Graig W. Smith, M.D.

COMMON PREGNANCY MYTHS

Fact or Folklore?

WOODVIEW
PUBLISHING

Published by Woodview Publishing
P.O. Box 31142
Cincinnati, OH 45231

Printed in the United States of America

Cataloging-in-Publication

Smith, Graig W.
Common pregnancy myths : fact or folklore? / Graig W. Smith. — 1st ed.
p. cm.
Includes bibliographical references and index.
ISBN: 0-9663664-2-5

1. Pregnancy. 2. Childbirth. I. Title.

RG525.S65 1998 618.2
QBI98-446

This book is dedicated to:

My wife, Janet, for all of her technical and personal support...

My three children, Ryan, Eric and Lindsay who encouraged me to write this book knowing it meant more time away from them...

All of my patients who shared their myths with me through the years.

Contents

Introduction

What on earth possessed me to write a book on pregnancy myths and facts? Let me answer this by telling you a little bit about myself and then by explaining my motives. I am an obstetrician from the Midwest who has been in private practice since 1985. Along with my private practice duties, I am on the teaching staff of a large Ohio hospital which trains OB/GYN residents and upper-year medical students. Throughout the course of my everyday work life, I am constantly hearing questions asked by residents, medical students, and patients in regard to pregnancy. One of my goals has been to prod the students and residents to think for themselves, instead of just parroting what some other more senior medical person tells them is true. If it were not for this type of critical thinking, we might still believe that the earth is flat or that life can be generated from inanimate objects. In regard to my patients, I enjoy discussing their questions and want to provide them with answers that are as helpful and accurate as possible. So my first reason for undertaking this task was to try to sort out fact from garbage and share this knowledge with those who come in contact with pregnant women as well as with the women themselves.

The second reason I decided to tackle this subject, and by far the most important, was quite simply to have some fun. As we go through our lives, we need a break from the harsh realities of everyday living. Sometimes when I am in the middle of a tough surgical case and an anesthesiologist or nurse tells a 30-second "joke of the day," the tension in the room starts to dissipate and many times I can get a new perspective on the situation. Likewise in life, we sometimes need to sit back, get a good chuckle, and forget about our problems for awhile. This book attempts to fulfill this need more than anything else.

I have to admit that I have a third motive for writing this book which is a little devious. No, it's not fame and fortune. Somehow I doubt that this book will get me too many nominations for a Pulitzer Prize. This motive can be explained best by an analogy—eating my favorite cookie—the Oreo. The outside is okay, but nothing beats that sweet, creamy inside. Well, buried inside this book are some concepts that I hope may bring some insight and comfort to someone's life. For example, I have run across women in my practice who have a great deal of guilt about something terrible they think they may have done during their pregnancy that resulted in a miscarriage. When I sit down with them and weed out the common myths related to miscarriage, many are overcome with relief to find out that their actions usually had nothing to do with their loss. It is as if a great weight has been lifted off their shoulders. Hopefully this book may act to rid some burdens of guilt that a few of you may be carrying around in regard to a previous pregnancy. Maybe it will also keep someone from propagating a hurtful myth.

The book is organized into six basic sections: I) Myths and Facts of Conception and Sex, 2) Myths and Facts of Labor, 3) Myths and Facts of Pregnancy Risks, 4) Myths and Facts of Pregnancy Loss, 5) Postpartum Myths and Facts, and 6) Miscellaneous Myths and Facts. These categories seemed to naturally fall out as I organized my thoughts. Within each category are several myths and facts in the form of questions and possible answers. After reading each question, take a guess at the answer. Then read the ANSWER section to see what my research has revealed. In some cases, the answers might surprise you, whereas others are a little more predictable. As you are reading through the book, you may think of your own questions. If you do, please write them down and send them to me. I will do my best to include them in my next edition. My mailing and e-mail addresses are included at the end of this introduction.

Finally, I would like to thank all of my patients and their family members who have contributed ideas for this book. If it were not for the grandmas and "Aunt Susies" of the world, the book would never have gotten off the ground. Throughout the course of my day, I come in contact with numerous patients, friends, and relatives who ask interesting and sometimes bizarre questions. Whenever a particularly interesting question is asked, I just jot it down. After accumulating a number of these, I start pouring over text books and journals at the local medical library along with tapping into the National Medical Library in Washington, D.C. through my personal computer. Two resources that have been particularly helpful to me are *Williams Obstetrics* by the folks at the University of Texas Southwestern in Dallas and *Maternal Fetal Medicine* by Creasy and Resnick. Both of these texts have been of great value to me in my career and are frequently referenced throughout the book.

Oh yes. Don't let me forget to mention my biggest fan and critic—my wife. Whenever I finish researching a particular subject, I have my wife review the material and make recommendations. Frequently her comments are, "What...are you crazy?" or "You aren't really going to put that in print are you?" I can always judge by the size of her smile or the raising of her eyebrows whether I have something interesting or provocative enough to include in my menagerie. Well, enough of this pregame wordiness—let's get on with our myths and facts.

Graig W. Smith, M.D.
P.O. Box 31142
Cincinnati, Ohio 45231

E-mail: graig@iglou.com

(Please notice that my name begins with a *G,* not a *C.* I mention this not because I am particularly sensitive about my name, but because this error will send your e-mail to the outer reaches of Mongolia and will deprive me of the pleasure of hearing from you)

Myths & Facts of Conception & Sex

I entitled this first section "MYTHS AND FACTS OF CONCEPTION AND SEX" mainly to get your attention early in the game. Whenever the word sex comes up, our heart rates tend to increase, our breathing gets a little faster, and our senses become a little more heightened. After all, our specie's interest in sex is what got us here in the first place and what will keep us here, hopefully for some time to come. The attraction of men and women and their propensity to bear children down through the ages has lead to the development of some real whopper myths *(and coincidentally keeps my children clothed and fed).*

These QUESTIONS deal with creating children *(which is certainly a lot more fun than raising them...at least when they hit the teenage years)* and predicting their gender before birth. Gender prediction is not as prevalent as it used to be before the advent of ultrasounds. Today, it is possible to know the sex of your child with virtual certainty long in advance of the big moment. Creating the sex that you want is another question. Well, before I lose your interest, let's proceed to MYTHS AND FACTS OF CONCEPTION AND SEX.

QUESTION: Is there anything I can do to increase the odds of getting pregnant in any given month?

A. Sure. A bottle of wine, a candlelight dinner, and some old Frank Sinatra records all around the middle of the cycle and you're all set.
B. Sure, but forget Sinatra. Go with some Smashing Pumpkins, a little massage oil, throw in a some handcuffs, and you've got a winner.
C. Yes. Your chances are increased only if you are under twenty, unmarried, and it's your first time.
D. Yes. Simply make a date every other day in the middle of the cycle, keep it simple, and your odds are pretty good.

ANSWER: D.

This is one of the most common questions I am asked throughout the course of a day. Why? Quite simply because we are planners. We want to time our pregnancies to fit exactly in certain niches in our lives. By the time you coordinate both of your work schedules, avoid being too far along when your sister-in-law gets married so you'll fit into that bridesmaid dress, and work around the ski trip to Colorado, it leaves little time to accomplish your goal. Because we are always under these time constraints, is there anything you can do to increase your odds of conceiving during one certain month or another?

First of all, you can figure out when it is that you are most likely to ovulate during any given month. Generally speaking, most women ovulate 14 days before the start of their next period or menstrual flow. The part of the cycle that varies from woman to woman is from the first day of bleeding to the time of ovulation. Let me make this a little more clear with some examples. If we call the first day of bleeding "day #1," and a woman has a perfect 28-day cycle, she will ovulate on day #14. If she has a 30-day cycle, she will ovulate on day #16. A 32-day cycle will yield an ovulation on day #18, and so on. So if your cycles are fairly regular, you can get a pretty good idea of when you are likely to ovulate by using this knowledge. Other more sophisticated techniques that are used to document ovulation are basal body temperature charts and ovulation predictor kits.

Basal body temperatures rely on the fact that a woman's body temperature rises slightly after ovulation. This rise is very small, however, and to pick up this subtle change, you must take your temperature first thing in the morning before you get out of bed. If you get out of bed to go to the bathroom or let the dog out, this activity generates enough heat to screw up the test. The biggest disadvantage of this test, however, is that it is retrospective. By this I mean that you don't know that you have ovulated until it has already occurred, and then it may be too late to conceive. Therefore basal body temperatures are used mainly to get an idea of when ovulation occurs so that this information can be used for future cycles. By using the 14-day rule that I explained earlier, though, you can predict the day of ovulation about as well as by using basal body temperatures.

Ovulation predictor kits became popular because they can *predict* when ovulation will occur. A woman figures out approximately when she will ovulate and then begins testing her urine a few days ahead of time. Chemicals are added to the urine samples each day which pick up a hormone surge that occurs 12 to 24 hours before ovulation. When a woman sees a certain color change, she knows that she is likely to ovulate within 12 to 24 hours. She then needs to explain to her husband's boss why she needs to pull him out of his stockholders' meeting in Maui in such an urgent fashion. The drawback of the test is that it is relatively expensive, and if a woman has irregular cycles, she may need to buy more than one kit per month.

Once you have figured out when you are likely to ovulate, the next logical question is "How often should you have intercourse?" Once a day? Once a week? Saturdays and holidays? Since most sperm are alive for a day or two and the egg is alive for a day or two, the optimum frequency of intercourse seems to be every other day in the middle of the cycle. If intercourse occurs too frequently, then the number of sperm per ejaculation take a dive and this affects conception negatively. If the Saturdays and holidays system is used, then intercourse may be so infrequent that the egg and sperm die an agonizing and unrequited death while never knowing the joy of each others' company *(Quite poetic, don't you think?)*. Anyway, every other day seems to fit the bill pretty well.

Something else to remember is that conception is really a numbers game. The idea is to get the greatest number of sperm around the egg at the time of ovulation. During intercourse, however, most of the semen containing the sperm runs out of the vagina. Therefore, don't jump out of bed right after intercourse. I tell my patients to simply place a small pillow under their hips for 15 or 20 minutes after intercourse, and this should serve to get the little fellas moving in the right direction. *(Despite a popular belief, standing on your head after intercourse might provide an interesting visual extravaganza for your partner, but really is quite unnecessary.)*

In summary, then, it seems that intercourse every other day in the middle of the cycle with slight hip elevation should theoretically increase your chances of conceiving in any given month. Save the trapeze for the remaining days of the cycle.

QUESTION: Can you really determine the sex of your baby by altering how you have intercourse.

A. No. It's always a 50/50 shot no matter how you're shooting.
B. There are ways to tip the scale, but these methods are mainly theoretical, fairly impractical, and may actually lead to a decreased fertility rate.
C. Sure. These sure-fire methods work pretty well and are guaranteed to spice up that boring Saturday night roll in the hay.
D. To find out this answer, you have to pick up a copy of my next book entitled "Making Love on the Bridges of Madison County: How To Determine the Sex of Your Baby by Choosing the Right Bridge."

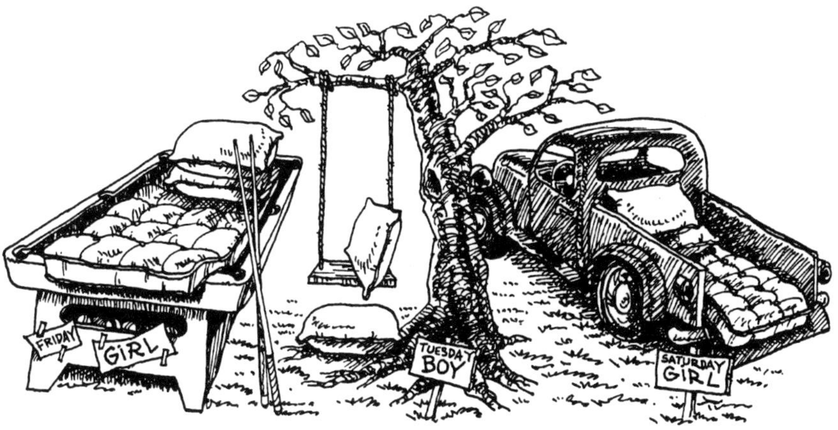

ANSWER: B.

Let me see...If you have intercourse on Wednesday during the full moon in your cousin Willie's pickup truck, does this assure a boy or a girl? I can't remember. Or maybe it's Tuesdays on your Aunt Susie's pool table. Whatever the theory, many books have been written about techniques that may be used to select the sex of your baby. For the most part, you are wasting your money by investing in this literature. Much of this advice is not well founded and may actually lead to a decrease in fertility by altering the frequency and timing of intercourse.

I was able to find one study that suggested that if intercourse occurs a day or two before ovulation then you will be more likely to have a boy. Likewise, intercourse right around the time of ovulation is more likely to yield a girl. The theory of why this happens goes like this: Boy sperm or Y sperm are 4 percent lighter than girl or X sperm. The Y sperm are also faster and live longer than their X counterparts. If intercourse occurs a day or two before ovulation, there are more of the longer living Y sperm around when ovulation actually occurs. If intercourse occurs close to the time of ovulation, the manly Y and wimpo X sperm have relatively equal numbers and an equal chance to reach the prize egg. Therefore this theory says that the farther away from ovulation you have intercourse, the greater the chance that you will have a boy. Intercourse right around the time of ovulation will yield equal chances of each. Remember, though, that the egg and the sperm have an average life of a day or two and that intercourse too far from ovulation may lead to no live sperm available to fertilize the egg for that cycle. This theory also has the disadvantage of only being able to increase your chances of having a boy. The experimenters also admit that these differences in sperm are slight and the number of people in the study are small, so their data is probably not very practical for the average couple.

If intercourse timing is not all that useful for trying to select out for boys or girls, then is there anything that really does work? There are separation techniques that are able to separate the X sperm from the Y sperm based on the difference in their weight. Once the X and Y sperm are separated, the sperm is then artificially inseminated into the woman. These techniques are not perfect, however, and yield a 75 percent chance of getting a boy when a boy is desired and a 69 percent chance of getting a girl when a girl is desired. Moreover the technique is too expensive and laborious to be of practical use today.

REFERENCES

Beernink FJ, Dmowski WP, Ericsson RJ. Sex preselection through albumin separation of sperm. *Fertil Steril* 1993 Feb; 59(2): 382-386.

France JT, Graham FM, Gosling L, Hair PI. A prospective study of the preselection of the sex of offspring by timing intercourse relative to ovulation. *Fertil Steril* 1984; 41(6): 894–900

Glass RH. Sex preselection. *Obstet Gynecol* 1977; 49(1): 122–126.

QUESTION: How long do you need to be off of birth control pills before becoming pregnant?

A. At least three months.
B. At least six months.
C. Preferably one year.
D. There is no need to wait at all.

ANSWER: D.

It is common knowledge that you need to be off of oral contraceptives for at least three months before becoming pregnant, right? At least that's what I was taught in my OB/GYN residency. Unfortunately, I was one of those residents who always asked "Why?" The most common answer I got was, "Because I told you so, kid...get off my back." The second most common response was, "Well, you have to get the pills out of your system or they will harm the baby." When I would further question my mentors on the subject of how and why this would be injurious to the pregnancy, I realized that this practice of waiting to become pregnant had been handed down through the years without much thought. It sounds reasonable, but is there really any basis for giving this advice?

In order to see if it is important to "get these drugs out of your system" prior to pregnancy, maybe we should see what happens to women who take oral contraceptives when they are already pregnant and don't realize it. Remember that the failure rate of oral contraceptives is around 1 percent. Since these women become pregnant while on the pills, their babies are exposed to the highest possible levels of these drugs. If you look at the babies born to these women compared to women who have never used birth control pills before, is there any difference in abnormalities in their children? Early studies in the 1960s and 1970s implied that there were increases in birth defects, especially of the heart, in children exposed to oral contraceptives. More recent studies used larger numbers of women and corrected for other variables such as maternal health, genetic risks, and other drug use. These studies showed that there is no increased risk of birth defects in the children of these women. I was also unable to find any increase in the miscarriage rate in women who conceive shortly after stopping oral contraceptives.

In my practice I advise couples who want to become pregnant to stop their birth control pills at the end of the pack and thenbegin trying to conceive as soon as they are ready. As a footnote, please also understand that even though oral contraceptives do not seem to cause problems when taken early in pregnancy, any woman who suspects that she may be pregnant while taking these pills should be tested and stop her pills if she is pregnant. It makes little sense to continue this medication if a failure has occurred.

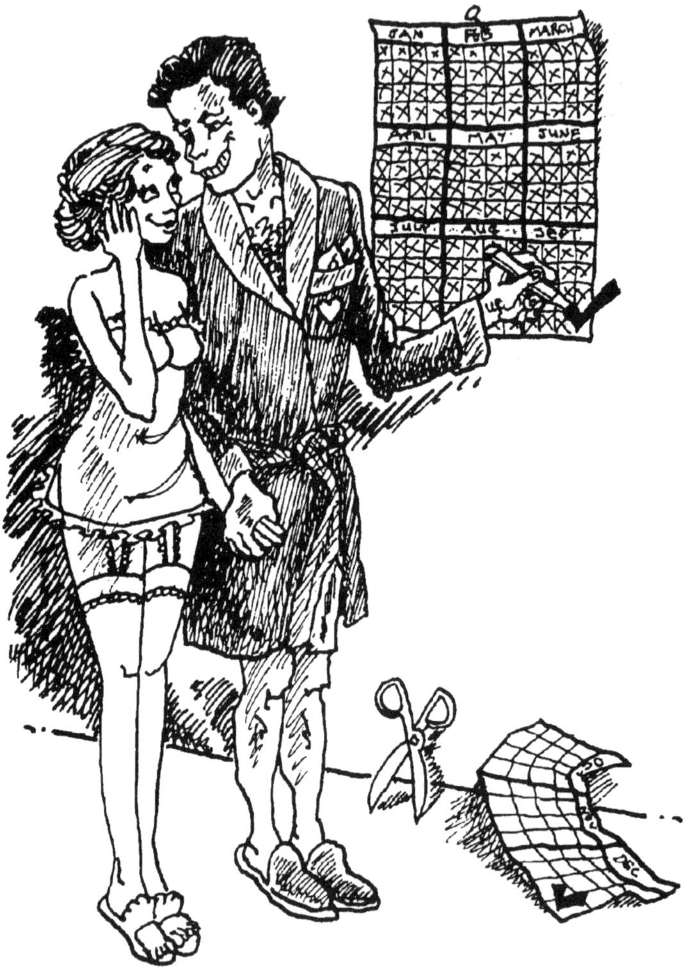

REFERENCES

Bracken MB. Oral contraceptives and congenital malformations in offspring: a review and meta-analysis of the prospective studies. *Obstet Gynecol* 1990 Sep; 76(3 pt 2): 552–7.

Harlap S, Shiono PH, Ramcharan S. Congenital abnormalities in the offspring of women who used oral and other contraceptives around the time of conception. *Int J Fertil* 1985; 30(2): 39–47.

QUESTION: Speaking of birth control pills, how do they actually work in preventing pregnancy?

A. By giving women frequent headaches and therefore reducing the frequency of intercourse.
B. By increasing mood swings in women and therefore reducing the frequency of intercourse.
C. By convincing a woman's body that she is already pregnant.
D. Nobody really knows.

ANSWER: C.

Birth control pills are based on the concept that pregnant women don't ovulate. It wouldn't make much sense for a woman who is already pregnant to continue to ovulate, would it? Well, the reason she doesn't ovulate is that during pregnancy, the placenta pours out large amounts of hormones which get into the bloodstream. The ovaries sense all of these hormones, decide that there are enough hormones around, and stop producing hormones of their own. Since the ovaries need their own hormones in order to ovulate, ovulation stops during pregnancy.

This lack of ovulation during pregnancy was noticed many years ago and someone got the bright idea of giving these hormones to women who were not pregnant in order to prevent pregnancy. They used two types of hormones: estrogen and progesterone. You will find these hormones in all of the standard birth control pills used today. Because these pills consist of different combinations of estrogen and progesterone, we call these pills combination oral contraceptives. A special type of birth control pill containing only progesterone (sometimes referred to as a "mini-pill") may be used for some women who don't tolerate estrogen well or women who can't use estrogen because they are breast feeding. The main drawback of this pill is that it is not as good at controlling bleeding as the combination pills.

The way oral contraceptives work is that a woman takes them daily for three weeks in order to create a "false pregnancy" and stop ovulation. During the fourth week of the cycle, a woman stops taking the pills (or she may take pills with no drugs in them to keep in the habit of taking something each day). During this week of "placebo" pills, there is a drop in the amount of hormone in the bloodstream and the inside lining of the uterus is sloughed off, leading to vaginal bleeding. We call this bleeding a "period," but it is very different from the bleeding that occurs during a menstrual cycle. During a menstrual cycle, ovulation takes place and if the egg is not fertilized, the lining of the uterus is sloughed. The main difference between normal menstrual bleeding and withdrawal bleeding from birth control pills is that there is no ovulation on birth control pills.

If all you are trying to do is avoid a pregnancy, why then, do women need to bleed once a month on birth control pills? The answer is simple...to make sure that they are not pregnant. Since there is a failure rate of around 1 percent on birth control pills, bleeding during the fourth week of pills assures a woman that she is not pregnant and allows her to proceed to the next pack. If a woman does not bleed on her last week of pills, it doesn't necessarily mean that she is pregnant, but that she should have a pregnancy test performed before starting her next pack.

Besides the obvious effect of providing birth control, oral contraceptives have the added benefit of reducing the amount of cramping and bleeding during periods, giving predictable cycles, and of possibly reducing the incidence of ovarian and uterine cancer. In fact, I have many women who continue using birth control pills even after tubal ligations just to control their cramping and bleeding. The most common side effects are similar to the symptoms that women experience during early pregnancy such as nausea, headaches, and breast tenderness. More severe side effects from birth control pills such as increased blood clotting are very rare, but should be considered before going on them. As a general rule, the vast majority of women do very well on birth control pills, and as long as a woman doesn't smoke and has reasonable cholesterol levels, using them all the way up until menopause is safe and effective.

QUESTION: Do your odds of getting pregnant and having a successful pregnancy decrease with age?

A. Yes, but only for women.
B. Yes, but only for men.
C. Yes. This is true for men and for women, but it affects men at a later age.
D. No, fertility remains fairly constant throughout a couple's lifetime.

ANSWER: C.

For women, pregnancy rates begin to decline around age 30 and significantly decline after age 40. This decreased rate is due to a number of factors including the following: 1) There is a decrease in normal ovulation with age. 2) Physical impairments of the reproductive organs increase with age. An example would be the increase in muscular tumors of the uterus called fibroids. These are usually benign but may distort the uterus and obstruct the tubes. 3) Genetic abnormalities of the infant increase with age. This also leads to an overall increase in miscarriages as many genetically abnormal fetuses are lost early in pregnancy. 4) Medical illnesses such as hypertension and diabetes increase with age and decrease fetal survival. Hypertension decreases blood flow to the placenta and diabetes increases fetal size making deliveries more difficult.

Even though my previous comments concerning fertility and age are true, these facts need to be placed in perspective. The odds of getting pregnant and having a normal labor and delivery resulting in a normal child may be excellent for any given couple whether they are in their twenties, thirties, or forties, if they are in reasonable health and have a reasonable lifestyle. The genetic risks as they relate to age are, in my opinion, greatly over exaggerated. Let me give you an example. Down's syndrome is well known to increase with age. The risk of a woman having a child with Down's syndrome at age 40 is roughly 1 in 100, or 1 percent. Although this is roughly ten times the risk for a woman in her mid-twenties (1 in 1000), there is about a 99 percent chance that her child will not have Down's syndrome. Pretty good odds if you are a betting kind of person. Most of the other types of genetic disorders that increase with age work in this fashion.

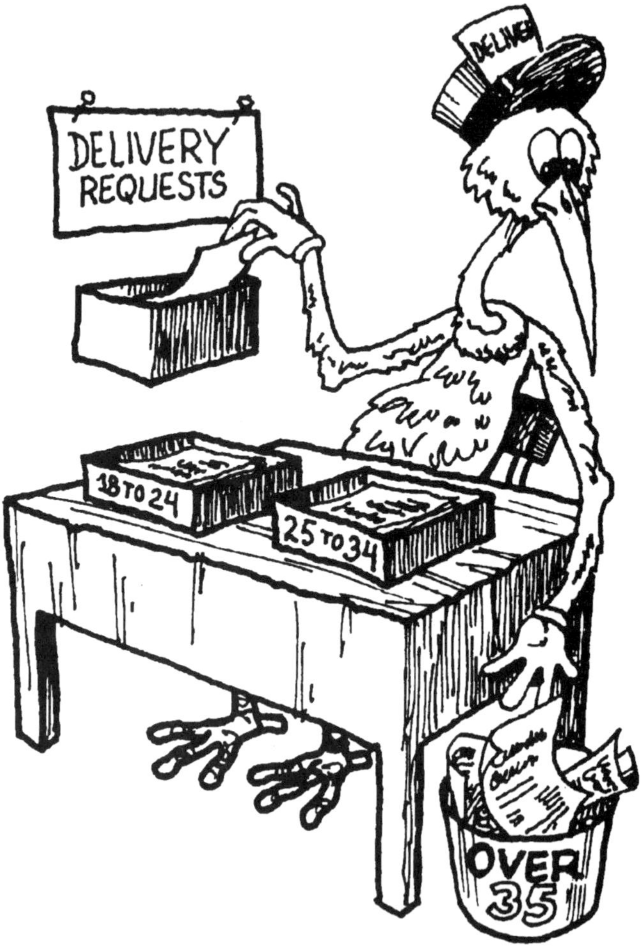

If what I just said is true, then why does everybody make a big deal about completing your family before the age of 35. Is there something magical about the age 35? Does everything fall apart after you reach this age? Not at all. If I may, please allow me to return to my Down's syndrome example that I used above to illustrate a point (Please forgive me for picking on Down's syndrome, but I know more about it than most other genetic conditions). As I stated, the incidence of Down's syndrome at age 25 is about 1 in 1000 and the incidence at age 40 is 1 in 100. If you look at this incidence at age 35, it is roughly 1 in 300. So what is the big deal about age 35? *Hold on to your pants...I'm getting to that part...*You must understand that genetic disorders may be detected by a procedure called amniocentesis. During this procedure, a needle is inserted into the uterus of a pregnant woman and fluid is withdrawn. This fluid contains fetal cells which tell us if a fetus is genetically normal or not. *Are you still with me?* This procedure is relatively safe, but like any procedure, there are risks of complications (such as injury to the fetus or miscarriage). This complication rate so happens to be about 1 in 300...the same as the risk of Down's syndrome at age 35. So before the age of 35, the risk of complications from amniocentesis is greater than the risk of having a child with Down's syndrome. At age 35 the risks are equal, and after age 35 the risk of having a child with Down's syndrome is greater than the risk of complications from amniocentesis. This is the only reason genetic testing is offered at age 35 and above—not because anything magical happens at this age.

In my practice, more and more couples are waiting until later in life to start a family. Even though genetic and medical risks are somewhat increased, the vast majority of these couples do very well. I frequently tell them that other factors such as diaper changing and late night infant care are much more important factors to weigh in their decision to have or not have children because these "risks" are 100 percent.

You may have noticed that I related the decrease in fertility to an increase in a woman's age but failed to comment about men. Although the frequency of intercourse decreases with age, overall male fertility doesn't decrease until about age 60. At this time the quality of the semen declines, leading to a drop in fertility rates.

REFERENCES

Berkowitz GS, Skovron ML, Lapinski RH, Berkowitz RL. Delayed childbearing and the outcome of pregnancy. *N Engl J Med* 1990; 332: 659–664

Cnattingius S, Forman MR, Berendes HW, Isotalo L. Delayed childbearing and risk of adverse perinatal outcome. *JAMA* 1992; 268: 886–890

Federation CECOS, Schwartz D, Mayaux MJ. Female fecundity as a function of age. *N Engl J Med* 1982; 306: 404–406

Friede A, Baldwin W, Rhodes PH, Buehler JW, Strauss LT. Older maternal age and infant mortality in the United States. *Obstet Gynecol* 1988; 72: 152–157

Hollander D, Breen JL. Pregnancy in the older gravida: how old is old? *Obstet Gynecol Surv* 1990; 45: 106–112

Prolog. *Reproductive Endocrinology.* Third edition. Critique Book. American College of Obstetrics and Gynecology. pp. 112–113

Stovall SW, Toma SK, Hammond MG, Talbert LM. The effect of age on female fecundity. *Obstet Gynecol* 1991; 77:33–66

QUESTION: If you exercise too much, can it keep you from getting pregnant?

A. Yes. Excessive exercise can keep you from ovulating, which is a definite setback in regard to becoming pregnant.
B. Yes, but only if your exercise involves moving a fork from your plate to your mouth.
C. Only if you're mid-cycle and your partner can't catch up with you.
D. No. Exercise is always beneficial and has no effect on fertility.

ANSWER: A.

With exercise, and just about anything else, too much of a good thing can be detrimental. Exercise is something our society could use more of, but taken to its extreme, it can effect fertility negatively. When female athletes are engaged in excessively strenuous activities, many of these athletes will stop ovulating and therefore stop having periods. What's the big deal, you might say? You could save a bundle on sanitary napkins, and what woman would miss a day of bleeding while negotiating a 10-K run? It's true that this lack of bleeding is an advantage in that it may allow for more comfortable competitions for some women. But if these same women decide to make that foray into motherhood, conception may be a bit difficult without the ability to ovulate. Exercise amenorrhea, as it is known medically, is a condition that strikes quite a few women in our progressively more health-conscious society. In my practice, the women who appear to be at most risk for this problem are dancers, gymnasts, and competitive runners.

There are two major factors that keep these women from ovulating. First of all, there seems to be a critical amount of body fat needed for a woman to ovulate. If a woman has an extremely low proportion of body fat, it can interfere with the production of estrogen, which is essential for ovulation. On the average, the competitive female athlete has about 50 percent less body fat than your average couch potato. This same decrease in body fat is seen in women suffering from anorexia nervosa. In fact, the most common reason women with anorexia nervosa come to the office for help is their lack of periods. The major difference between athletes and women with anorexia nervosa is that the athlete maintains good muscle mass and has a solid grasp on what she is doing to her body. The patient with anorexia nervosa has a distorted body image and sees herself as overweight even in the face of emaciation.

The second reason female athletes may not ovulate stems from a stress-induced suppression of areas within the brain that are necessary for ovulation. This is especially apparent in dancers, gymnasts, or runners whose lives revolve around strenuous daily practice routines that demand physical and mental perfection. An example of how stress affects ovulation can be seen in my patient population. My office is next to the University of Cincinnati, and around exam time I often see female students who have skipped periods and are afraid they might be pregnant. Sometimes they are right, but many times the stress of their exams has kept them from ovulating. Once exams are over and life returns to normal, their menstrual patterns usually return. In some athletes, the effect of stress may be combined with decreased body fat making conception virtually impossible without some type of intervention.

Can anything be done to overcome these factors in athletes who desire to become pregnant? One obvious solution is for these women to back off on their exercise program to the point where ovulation is possible. Until recently, this was all we had to offer for this problem. Many women, however, consider their exercise an integral part of their lives and want to maintain their training while trying to conceive and even throughout much of their pregnancy. Fortunately today, with the onset of modern fertility techniques, medication may be used to allow ovulation in the face of continued exercise. These medicines may be given orally each cycle or injected daily until ovulation occurs.

Another effect of strenuous exercise on the female body that should not be overlooked is the loss of bone mass these women may get in response to their low estrogen levels. This bone loss is similar to the loss postmenopausal women experience and may lead to the development of osteoporosis. If left unchecked, this bone loss can cause career-ending bone fractures. Therefore competitive athletes may need to be placed on extra estrogen (similar to the estrogen replacement therapy given to postmenopausal women) to maintain their bone integrity and avoid these fractures.

So forget the exercise and blimp out a little. Enjoy that ice cream sundae for dessert tonight knowing that you are doing your part to propagate your fertility and maintain your bone density.

REFERENCES

Speroff L, Glass RH, Kase NG. *Clinical Gynecologic Endocrinology and Infertility.* Fifth edition. Williams & Wilkins. Baltimore, Maryland. pp. 438–41, 1994.

QUESTION: Are "test tube" babies different from "naturally conceived" babies?

A. Yes. They are longer and thinner than other babies due to their cramped living quarters.

B. Their appearance is no different, but their early growth is slower due to space confinements.

C. They are the same except that nobody knows who their true parents are.

D. There is absolutely no difference in the appearance of these children. They vary only in how they were conceived.

ANSWER: D.

So-called "test tube" babies are children who are conceived through a process known as in vitro fertilization. The term "test tube" baby is a rather derogatory one and is actually incorrect. The term conjures up visions of tiny babies growing up in glass cylinders until someone comes along and releases them into the arms of their parents à la Thumbelina. There are actually no test tubes used and the whole process acts to assist a couple in conceiving rather than totally replacing them. Let me explain.

In vitro fertilization (or IVF for short) is a procedure in which eggs from the mother and sperm from the father are brought together in a glass dish where the eggs are fertilized. These fertilized eggs are then inserted through the cervix where they implant on the surface of the uterus and grow. This process was devised back in the 1970s, and in 1978 Drs. Steptoe and Edwards reported the first IVF birth in England. Originally, it was used to help couples conceive when women had fallopian tube damage that prevented the egg and sperm from finding each other. Today, there are multiple centers using this technique to assist couples who are infertile due to poor sperm quality, endometriosis, sperm antibodies (proteins that a woman produces that destroy sperm), and those with unexplained infertility.

The process is started by giving a woman hormones that allow her to produce a number of mature eggs at once. These eggs are then surgically removed and placed into a special growth medium. Sperm is then obtained from the father *(using the magazine-hand-cup technique)* and placed into the growth medium with the eggs. Fertilization of these eggs usually occurs within 24 hours. Once the eggs have been fertilized, they begin to divide and by 48 hours or so they are ready to be placed into the uterus. So you see, the total out-of-body experience for these cells lasts about two days. The cells are then sucked up into a tiny straw-like instrument and inserted through the cervix and into the uterus. As many as four or five eggs are used to ensure that at least one will become fertilized and implant. If any are left over, they are frozen for use at a later time.

In a successful IVF program, the "take-home-baby rate" is in the neighborhood of 35 percent for women 36 years old and younger. For women over 36, the rate drops to around 10 percent. The success rate not only depends on age, but also on the number of cycles used. As an example, a group from Norfolk, Virginia, reports pregnancy rates that vary from 13.5 percent after one cycle to 57.8 percent after six cycles. In terms of complications, the biggest drawback of this procedure is the expense. Costs are in the range of a few thousand dollars per cycle, and as I mentioned above, a number of cycles may be required for a successful outcome. Another factor which may be viewed as negative is the multiple pregnancy rate which is around 30 percent (25 percent twins and 5 percent triplets or more). Consequently, couples using this technique should be prepared to author their own rendition of *Cheaper By the Dozen* if the embryo fairy decides to bless them with super-eggs that "just say yes" to their new found home.

Obviously, this procedure involves more finesse than a back yard tumble in the hay. That's why it should only be performed by centers with highly qualified personnel and the right technology. For the individual couple, it requires dedication and a lot of bucks and can place a tremendous strain on any couple both financially and emotionally. The end product, however, is no different than a child conceived in the back of a Chevy truck *(although a lot less fun)*. Overall, the procedure has given a great deal of joy to many couples who otherwise would have been childless.

REFERENCES

Speroff L, Glass RH, Kase NG. *Clinical Gynecologic Endocrinology and Infertility*. Fifth Edition. Williams & Wilkins Publ Co. Baltimore, Maryland. pp. 931-63, 1994.

QUESTION: Can you predict the sex of a baby before delivery by counting the fetal heart rate?

A. Yes. This method is actually more accurate than ultrasounds.
B. Yes, but the accuracy is only about 75 percent.

C. Yes, but the accuracy is only slightly greater than 50/50.

D. You can predict all you want, but the odds of predicting correctly are still 50/50.

ANSWER: D.

It was her second visit to the office and Mary Jones (not her real name...I just hate it when people always use the name "Smith" when they are quoting examples) brought her whole family to the office to hear the baby's heartbeat. She was 12 weeks along so that the little bambino's heartbeat should be picked up pretty easily. I said she brought her family but that was actually an understatement. She brought her two children ages one and three, her mother, her mother-in-law, her grandmother, and her husband. They filed into the exam room in a never-ending line. Her husband lagged far behind as he was weighted down with a diaper bag the size of Kansas, everyone else's coats, and an oversized bag of Cheerios, which was steadily being emptied into the two screaming siblings.

I followed the trail of Cheerios to the door of the exam room and squeezed in. After making the appropriate introductions to the extended family, I grabbed a bottle of ultrasound gel and squeezed a cold glob onto her mildly protuberant abdomen. After Mary's initial squeal from the cold jelly (that's one way we obstetricians get our kicks throughout the day—by torturing patients with cold ultrasound gel. Actually we tried warming the gel in the microwave once. After blowing up a couple of bottles, we quit) the steady fetal heart rate was heard. Tears started to flow...from me actually as one of the kids got tired of his Cheerios and bit into my ankle. Just about that time Grandma piped up, "Well, Doc, what is it...a boy or a girl?"

This scene occurs over and over again throughout the course of a day. It occurs so often that you begin to wonder if just maybe there is something to this cockeyed notion that you can predict a baby's sex by the heartbeat. It was this curiosity that led me to research this topic and come up with the following facts.

First of all, the most widely held notion in my practice is that girls are supposed to have faster heartbeats than boys. How this tale first got started nobody seems to know. In 1969 Dr. Brian Mabbott, a senior house officer in Northumberland, England saw this fact stated in a textbook and noticed that no references were given. He did a literature search and found no studies to support the theory of predicting a baby's sex using the heart rate. Dr. Mabbott proceeded to look up the records of 267 patients and write down the fetal heart rates of these patients when they were in labor. Heart rates were taken every half hour in the first stage of labor. (The first stage of labor is the time from the onset of labor until the patient is completely dilated and ready to start pushing). He also wrote down if the patient had a boy or a girl. Low and behold, he found that boys had a mean heart rate of 137, and for girls it was 142. This was a significant difference and therefore the idea sprang up that babies with heart rates over 140 were girls, and those with heart rates less than 140 were boys.

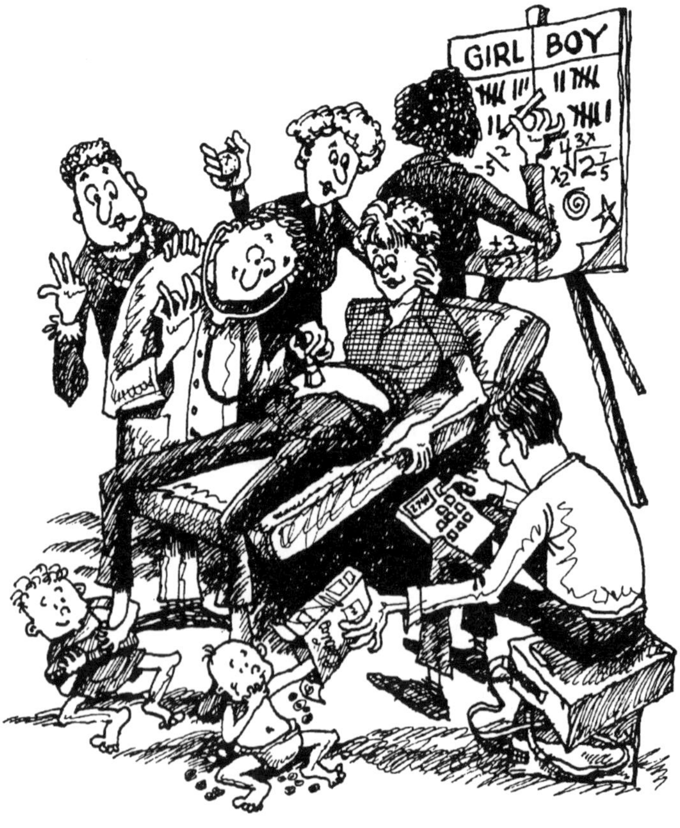

When you look at Dr. Mabbott's work in a little more detail, you can see that there are a few problems with his conclusions. First of all, fetal monitors were not commonly used back then. Fetal heart rates were approximated by listening with a stethoscope. Some nurses listened for 30 seconds and multiplied by two to get the heart rate per minute; other nurses listened for a full 60 seconds. This obviously introduced a great deal of error in the final calculations. The second problem is that these heart rates were recorded in the first stage of labor—not prior to labor when most patients want to know the sex. If a couple makes it to the first stage of labor without knowing the sex of their baby, they probably don't mind waiting a few more hours to find out at delivery.

Three studies were done after Dr. Mabbott's work that contradicted his findings: In 1986, Dr. Maurice Druzin et. al. from New York studied 37 pregnant patients from 19 to 40 weeks. Over 360 heart rate tests were done during this time using external fetal heart rate monitors. He found no differences between the heart rates of boys and girls. A radiologist from Austin, Texas used ultrasounds to compare heart rates to fetal sex in 1988 and found no correlation. Likewise, an OB/GYN nurse practitioner from Colorado Springs looked at 233 pregnancies and found that overall, boys weighed significantly more than girls. She then hypothesized that if small animals have faster heart rates than large animals (for instance a three gram shrew has a heart rate of 600 beats per minute versus an elephant with a heart rate of 25), then girls' hearts should beat faster than boys'. Her data, however, showed that the rates differed by an insignificant one beat per minute.

*But alas!...Don't despair grandma!...Hold on Aunt Susie!...*I was able to find a 1993 study from the University of Kentucky that gives a flicker of hope to those who propagate this myth. These researchers took the fetal heart rates of 128 women on each prenatal visit up to 32 weeks. A male sex was assigned to the fetus at 32 weeks if the heart rate was less than 140 beats per minute, and females were assigned for rates greater than 140. At delivery they found that they predicted a boy right 91 percent of the time and they were correct for girls 74 percent of the time. Just when it appears that we can wipe this myth off of the face of the earth, these guys gum up the works. As far as I am concerned, they need to be tied up and forced to eat Cheerios from the gooey hands of preschoolers for a week.

REFERENCES

Coughlin LL. Do fetal heart rates predict gender? [letter] J *Obstet Gynecol Neonatal Nurs.* 1993 Mar–Apr; 22(2): 105.

Druzin ML, Hutson JM, Edersheim TG. Relationship of baseline fetal heart rate to gestational age and fetal sex. *Am J Obstet Gynecol* 1986; 154: 1102–3.

DuBose TJ, Dickey D, Butschek CM, Porter P, Hill LW, Poole EK. [letter to the editor]. *J Ultrasound Med* 1988 7: 237–8.

Hall S, King K, Cox SM. Fetal sex prediction: the heart of the matter [letter]. *J Ky Med Assoc.* 1993 Sep; 91(9): 409–10.

Mabbott BJ. Comparison of the heart rate of the male and female foetus. *Br J Coin Pract.* 1969 Nov; 23(11); 447–8.

QUESTION: Are boys and girls born at an equal rate?

A. Boys are born at a higher rate.
B. Trick question—the rates are equal.
C. Girls are hardier at birth as well as later in life and therefore always outnumber the guys.
D. Nobody knows. Have you ever tried counting all of those newborns?...What a task!

ANSWER: A.

Surprisingly, boys and girls are not born at equal rates. Worldwide, there are about 105 boys born for every 100 girls. Overall, however, there are more females in the world since the life expectancy of women is longer than for men. Also of interest, there are at least two factors that seem to change the male/female birth ratio: 1) If ovulation drugs are used to conceive, this results in a slightly higher ratio of females. 2) Artificial insemination (placing previously ejaculated semen into the vagina or uterus) leads to a slightly higher ratio of males.

If you are wondering why the above facts are true...well...so am I. These facts fall into the "interesting but not yet explainable" category. But please, before you go out and buy that long-handled turkey baster, keep in mind that even though ovulation drugs and artificial insemination change the sex ratio, this difference is very small and of little practical importance to the average couple.

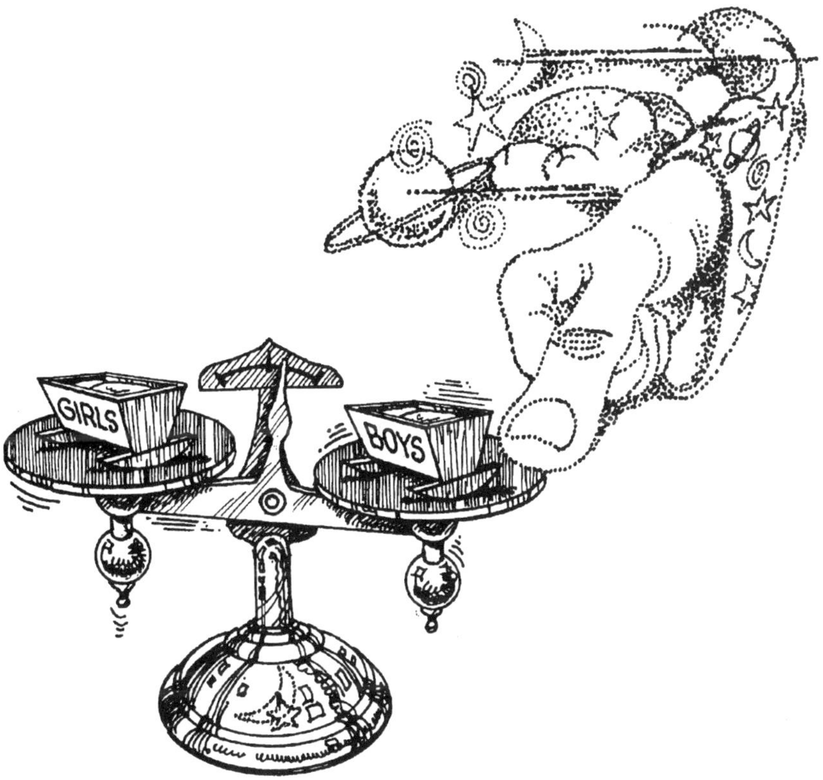

REFERENCES

Ericsson R J, Beernink F. Sex chromosome ratios in human sperm [letter]. *Fertil Steril* 1987; 47(3): 531–532.

Prolog: *Reproductive Endocrinology and Infertility.* Second edition. Critique Book. American College of Obstetrics and Gynecology. pp. 28–29.

Myths & Facts of Labor

As you might guess, one of the most common questions I am asked throughout the course of a day is, "When is this baby going to get here?" Unfortunately, my profession is a rather inexact science. I generally can narrow the range of an expected delivery to plus or minus two weeks, but even this range is only an educated guess. It's only natural for women to devise methods to try to predict their deliveries or possibly bring labor on. Do some of these methods actually work? Well…read on.

QUESTION: Does intercourse during pregnancy lead to premature labor?

A. Yes, but I have been sworn to an oath of secrecy by a lot of you guys out there not to reveal this devastating information.
B. Only when a trapeze is involved.
C. For the average pregnancy, probably not, but women at high risk of premature labor should keep it to a minimum.
D. There is no evidence—theoretical or actual—that links intercourse with initiating labor.

ANSWER: C.

No doubt there are many guys out there who are breathlessly awaiting my response to this question. This subject either comes up or is on the minds of virtually every couple (or at least the male member of the couple) who come in for their first prenatal visit. On occasion I forget to bring up the subject, but before the couple leaves the office the guy usually gets a sheepish look on his face and says, "Hey Doc, there is one more thing...uh...you know...when it comes to...a...you know...doing it...a..." And then I break in and say, "Oh yes, I forgot one important topic. As far as intercourse during pregnancy...," and I proceed to tell them a synopsis of the following.

Two early studies from the 1970s implied that there was at least a theoretical relationship between intercourse and preterm labor (labor before 8 ½ months). Most pregnant women will tell you that during intercourse and for a while afterward, they have contractions. If orgasm is reached, these contractions are even more pronounced. Actually these contractions occur in non-pregnant women also and are part of what a woman perceives as an orgasm. *(If this is true, you would think that labor would be an orgasmic experience...for some reason most of my patients don't describe their labor in quite that way.)* One of the reasons that these contractions occur is that the semen released during intercourse contains substances called prostaglandins. These prostaglandins lead directly to contractions of the uterus. (Sometimes prostaglandins are used to initiate labor in a woman who is overdue or in someone who needs to be delivered due to some problem in her pregnancy.) Theoretically, these prostaglandins may increase uterine activity in a pregnant woman who is at risk for premature delivery and therefore could increase her risk for delivering prematurely.

A second reason given for avoiding intercourse during pregnancy is the possibility of increased uterine infections leading to premature labor. By introducing new bacterial organisms into the vagina and cervix or by moving existing vaginal organisms into the cervix, these bacteria could cause an inflammation of the membranes surrounding the baby and cause a woman to go into labor.

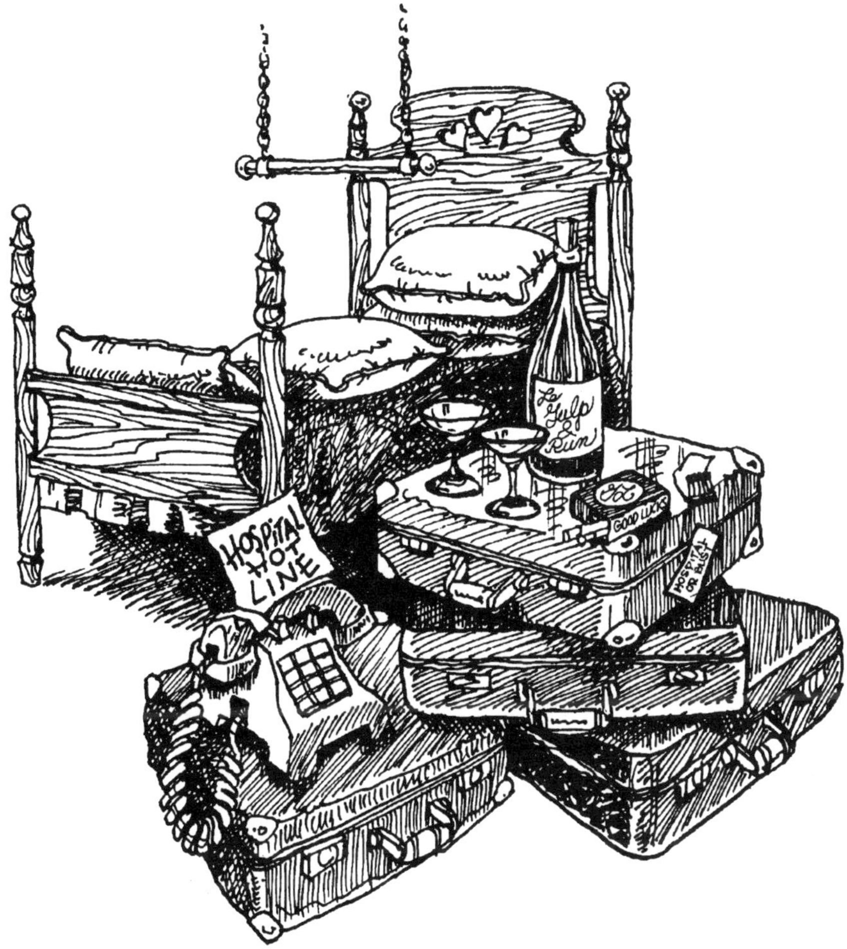

The increased uterine activity and the possibility of uterine infections has led some health care providers to restrict intercourse during pregnancy. Is there really any basis for doing this? Actually there have been studies looking at women who are at high risk for going into labor prematurely as well as low-risk women, and there seems to be little if any benefit in restricting intercourse in either group. An example of one such study is Neilson and Mutambira's research from Zimbabwe which was published in 1989. They looked at 126 women with twin pregnancies to see if the frequency of intercourse affected how long they were able to carry their pregnancy. Women with twins are at higher risk of going into labor prematurely than a singleton pregnancy. Early in the seventh month, 40 percent of these women were having intercourse, and this dropped to 24 percent by the ninth month. If those women who continued to have intercourse are compared to those women who stopped having intercourse, there is no difference in the rate of premature labor. So there you have it. The real challenge is not whether it is okay to have intercourse during pregnancy, but how to get close enough with that protuberant belly to make it happen. Before I leave this subject, however, I want to include a small disclaimer that if a woman has had a history of premature deliveries, a modest decrease in your merrymaking is not totally unreasonable based on the above theoretical considerations. That ought to keep you guys in line just a little.

REFERENCES

Creasy RK, Resnik R. *Maternal Fetal Medicine, Principles and Practice.* Third edition. W B Saunders. 1994:500.

Goodlin RC, Keller DW, Raffin M. Orgasm during late pregnancy and possible deleterious effects. *Obstet Gynecol* 38:916, 1971.

Naey RL. Coitus and associated amniotic fluid infections. *N Engl J Med* 301:1198, 1979.

Neilson JP, Mutambira M. Coitus, twin pregnancy, and preterm labor. *Am J Obstet Gynecol* 1989 Feb; 160(2): 416–8.

Wagner NN, Butler JC, Sanders JP. Prematurity and orgasmic coitus during pregnancy: Data on a small sample. *Fertil Steril* 27: 911, 1976.

QUESTION: Will drinking castor oil put a pregnant woman into labor?

A. Yes, and it is guaranteed to reduce a woman's time in labor by half.

B. Yes, but stand back because the explosion that results propels more than the baby into the waiting arms of the hapless obstetrician or midwife.

C. Probably not.

D. No, and there is actually some evidence that castor oil may have a harmful effect on the delivery.

ANSWER: D.

When a woman reaches those last few weeks of pregnancy, life can become pretty miserable. Trouble sleeping, shortness of breath, low back pain, and monumental mood swings are the hallmarks of this time. My guess is that since the beginning of time, pregnant women (and their partners) have been looking for a magical potion to send women into labor and put an end to this suffering.

Many years ago, someone realized that chugging down a putrid, slimy oil from the seed of a large African plant led to diarrhea like no tomorrow. The next logical thought was, "Gee, if castor oil empties out the bowel so well, what effect would it have on emptying out the uterus (i.e. labor) in a pregnant woman?" Logical question, huh?...NOT!...The gastrointestinal tract and the reproductive tract are two separate systems. Just because the bowel is jolted into overdrive by this liquid TNT, you should not expect the uterus to give a diddly darn. Moreover, if you do happen to go into labor, your helpless obstetrician or midwife will be on the receiving end of a tidal wave of do-do at the time of delivery.

Okay...Okay...I have to admit that there is one study that may keep this smelly myth alive (much to the chagrin of many deliverers of babies). In 1984 Lorna Davis, a certified midwife, took 196 pregnant women with ruptured membranes around their due date who were not in labor and divided them into two groups. One group was given two ounces of castor oil and the other group was given nothing. Within 24 hours, 75 percent of the castor oil group were in labor compared to 58 percent of the other group. The obvious problem with this study is that it deals with women with ruptured membranes. Most women who are contemplating using castor oil have intact membranes, and I found no study that showed any benefit in this group of women. Moreover, there may be some potential harm with using castor oil in pregnancy. In 1987 Mitri et. al. from South Africa suggested that not only do women who consume castor oil have diarrhea of gargantuan proportions, but so do their kids. They found that babies born to women who took castor oil prior to labor had a greater incidence of meconium-stained amniotic fluid. This greenish fluid results when the baby passes stool into the surrounding amniotic fluid and may result in fetal respiratory problems if the infant inhales this fluid at delivery. It also gives the kid an initial appearance somewhat akin to Kermit The Frog. Fortunately, the respiratory problems can usually be prevented by suctioning the infant's nose and mouth at delivery and the greenish hue washes off, but the tendency to hop around the crib may remain. *(Just kidding...Don't get so serious on me!)*

To summarize, do your local OB/midwife a favor...Ixnay on the astor oil cay. It will make him or her a happy camper, and you will be doing your part for frog population control.

REFERENCES

Davis L. The use of castor oil to stimulate labor in patients with premature rupture of membranes. *J Nurse Midwifery* 1984 Nov–Dec; 29(6):366–70.

Mitri F, Hofmeyr GJ, can Gelderen CJ. Meconium during labour—self-medication and other associations. *S Afr Med J* 1987 Apr 4; 71(7): 431–3.

QUESTION: Can stimulation of the breasts make a pregnant woman go into labor?

A. Yes. Breast stimulation causes uterine contractions that may lead to labor and therefore is recommended for women around their due date who want to go into labor.

B. Yes, but the stimulation may lead to contractions which are too frequent or severe and it is not recommended for "home use."

C. No. breast stimulation has nothing to do with uterine contractions.

D. There is no evidence one way or the other as to the effect of breast stimulation on contractions.

ANSWER: B.

One of the most commonly asked questions by pregnant women approaching their due date is, "What can I do to start labor?" Numerous "techniques" have been tried including drinking castor oil, power walking, or intercourse. Something physicians noticed long ago was that when a baby nurses, there is a reflex (called the letdown reflex) that causes something called oxytocin to be released from an area in the brain into the bloodstream. This oxytocin then travels to the breasts and causes small muscles in the nipples to contract and squirt milk into the hungry fella's mouth. When this oxytocin enters the bloodstream, it also travels to other regions of the body and one of these regions is the uterus. As this hormone reaches the uterus, contractions are initiated. These contractions keep the uterus from bleeding after delivery. This same hormone has actually been made synthetically under the brand name Pitocin and is used to initiate and maintain labor in some women.

During my residency in the early 1980s, we used nipple stimulation as a test to make sure a baby was doing okay. Warm, moist wash cloths were placed across a pregnant woman's breasts, and she was asked to stimulate her nipples enough to produce regular uterine contractions. The baby's heart rate was recorded while this was going on and if there was no drop in the heart rate, the baby was said to be okay. If decelerations of the heart rate were seen, then it was a sign that the baby wasn't all that happy and he (or she) was delivered. Today, this technique is not used as commonly for three main reasons. First of all, cases have been reported where the uterus is sensitive to this stimulation and becomes hyper-stimulated. When this occurs, the uterus clamps down around the baby for a prolonged period of time which decreases blood flow through the umbilical cord. Because blood flow is suddenly decreased to the baby, immediate delivery by Cesarean section is needed. A second reason for backing off on this technique is that it tends to be rather embarrassing for the mother as well as other personnel in the room. Although we tried to surround Mom with females to lessen the embarrassment, it was still somewhat difficult to have a woman rub her breasts appropriately to get the desired contractions. Lastly, there are other ways of evaluating the well-being of a baby utilizing less invasive means such as ultrasound.

REFERENCES

Creasy RK, Resnik R. *Maternal Fetal Medicine.* Third edition. WB Saunders Co. Phila., Pa. p. 323, 1994.

Huddleston JF, Sutliff G, Robinson D. Contraction stress test by intermittent nipple stimulation. *Obstet Gynecol* 63: 669, 1984.

Cunningham FG, MacDonald PC, Gant NF, Leveno KJ, Gilstrap LC. *Williams Obstetrics.* 19th edition. Appleton & Lange. Norwalk, Conn. p.1035, 1993.

Schellpfeffer MA, Hoyle D, Johnson JWC. Antepartal uterine hypercontractility secondary to nipple stimulation. *Obstet Gynecol* 65: 588, 1985.

QUESTION: If the baby "drops" or you lose your mucous plug, does it mean that labor will start soon?

A. Yes. If either one of these events happens, you should get to the hospital pronto.
B. No. Just put the baby back, locate your plug, and get back to bed.
C. No. Both of these events can happen minutes or weeks before labor starts.
D. Neither of these events ever occur in pregnancy.

ANSWER: C.

Ring! Ring! I rolled over in bed and grabbed the phone receiver off of the nightstand. It was 3 A.M. and I had just arrived home two hours earlier from the hospital and had fallen into a deep sleep. "Hello," I said in a scratchy, half-awake voice. "Hello, Dr. Smith. This is your answering service and we have a call from Mrs. Jones (the name has been changed to protect the guilty). Can we connect her through to you?" "Sure," I said.

"Hello, Dr. Smith. This is Lula Jones and I have just lost my mucous plug." After inquiring whether she was having any other symptoms such

as contractions or leaking fluid (which she was not), I told her that this was common during the end of pregnancy but not necessarily a sign of labor. After reassuring her that her call was not frivolous, I told her that it was nice hearing from her and that I would see her for her regular appointment later that day.

Losing the mucous plug refers to a blood-tinged mucous discharge that some women get late in their pregnancy. On the average, this occurs a few days before labor, but there is a great deal of variance. Some women may have this happen immediately before the onset of labor, while other women never have it happen at all. Therefore the news-breaking discovery that shattered my beauty sleep was fairly inconsequential. In all fairness to Mrs. Jones, she did the right thing by contacting me about an event that was new and had her concerned.

Later that day, Mrs. Jones showed up for her appointment with her mother. As I walked into the room, her mother quickly said, "Lula has really dropped. Does this mean that she should get her bags packed for the hospital?" "Not just yet," I said. "She is a few weeks away from her due date so don't get your hopes up." Is "dropping" of the baby or "lightening," as it is medically known, really a sign of impending labor? Actually it fits into the same category as mucous plugs. Many women will tell you that late in pregnancy they are suddenly able to breathe more easily and also feel an increase in pelvic pressure. These symptoms are due to the descent of the baby's head into the pelvis as well as an overall reduction of fluid around the baby. Just as in the case of mucous plugs, lightening happens shortly before the start of labor on the average, but is also variable. Some women experience it right before labor, some weeks before, and some never at all. Whatever the case, try to not get too excited about mucous plugs or dropping babies—especially at 3 A.M.

REFERENCES

Cunningham FG, MacDonald PC, Gant NF, Leveno KJ, Gilstrap LC: *Williams Obstetrics*. 19th edition. Appleton & Lange Norwalk, Conn. p. 340, 1993.

QUESTION: Are there more babies born during the full moon?

A. Definitely.
B. Only in less developed countries where births are not manipulated as much as in the U.S.
C. No, but those babies that are born during the full moon tend to be hairier and have a peculiar howl that sets them apart from most other babies.
D. Full moons have more to do with conception than birth.

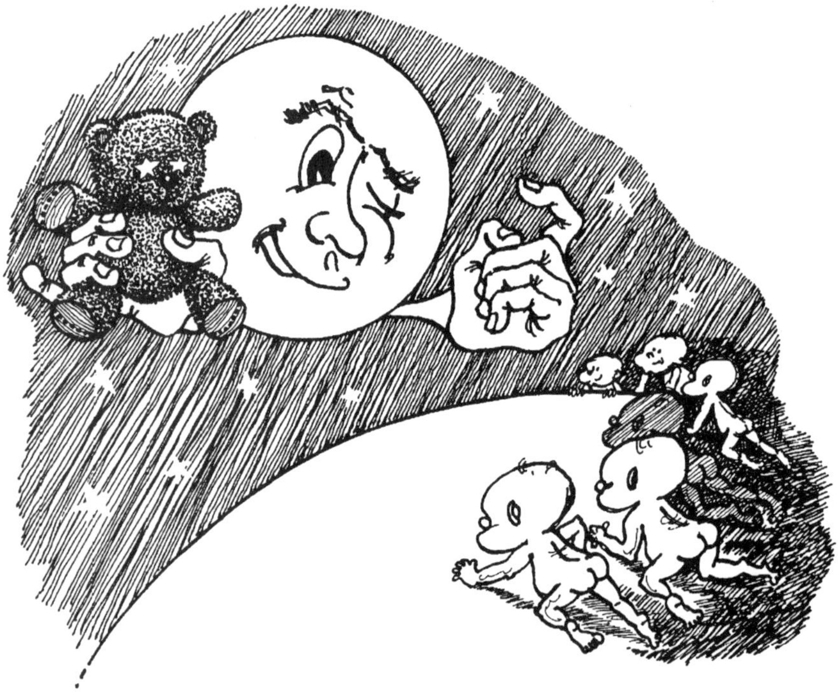

ANSWER: D.

I just finished delivering my fifth baby in the last twenty four hours and passed a group of nurses in the hall of a local hospital. It was 6:30 A.M. and the day-shift nurses were coming into the labor and delivery unit. I must have looked pretty haggard as one of them said, "Rough night, huh?"

"Pretty rough," I replied.

Another nurse spoke up, "Well, you could have predicted all those deliveries...It's the full moon, you know." The other nurses around her nodded in agreement and moved on.

This concept of the fluctuation of deliveries depending on the lunar cycle is commonly believed by ordinary folks as well as professionals. After my encounter with the above nurses, I began to think back about my own delivery experiences. There were many busy nights in labor and delivery when I would look out the window and sure enough, there was a full moon. Could it really be true that lunar cycles have some influence on deliveries?

Two recent studies from Italy and Mozambique have looked at over 13,000 births and have seen no correlation between those births and the lunar cycle. You may wonder why I refer only to studies outside of the United States. The reason is simple. Here in the U.S., we tend to manipulate our deliveries to a greater degree than in other countries. For example, we may induce women who go past their due date and stop the labor of women who are in danger of delivering early. Since we have smaller numbers of uninterrupted deliveries, these studies are harder to generate. At any rate, many children are undoubtedly conceived in the light of the moon, but deliveries seem to be a random event.

REFERENCES

Periti E, Biagotti R. Lunar phases and incidence of spontaneous deliveries. Our experience. *Minerva Gynecol* 1994 Jul–Aug; 46(7-8): 429–33.

Strolego F, Gigli C, Bugalgo A. The influence of lunar phases on the frequency of deliveries. *Minerva Gynecol* 1991 Jul–Aug; 43(78): 359–6.

QUESTION: Can storms bring on labor in pregnant women?

A. Yes. There is a direct correlation between falling barometric pressure and the onset of labor.
B. There is an increase in ruptured membranes when the barometer falls just prior to a storm, but no direct increase in actual labor.

C. Storms (especially snowstorms) have no effect on labor or membranes, but do act to bring people together and create more babies.

D. No studies have been done to answer this question one way or the other.

ANSWER: B.

It was 8 A.M. on a Saturday morning in February. I awoke suddenly to the sounds of our three children screaming, "Mom, Dad! Look outside!" I rolled out of bed, wiped the sleep from my eyes, trudged over to the window, and opened the blinds. Immediately the room was filled with a blazing white light. Indeed our yard looked like a Winter Wonderland. There must have been at least a foot of snow on the ground and it was still coming down.

"Can we go sled riding?" they chimed in harmony. "Can we, please?"

"Sure," I said. Let's get some breakfast and we'll head out to our favorite hill." Beep Beep Beep Beep! my pager squawked. I picked up the phone and called the answering service.

"Two patients just called and it looks like they're in labor," the operator said. "Must be due to the storm," she continued. "Our phones have been ringing off of the hook." I hung up and gathered the kids around.

"Tell you what guys, why don't you watch some cartoons and we'll do our sledding later today."

"Okay, Dad," they answered and headed off to the family room. As I started to dial the phone numbers of the patients, I thought, "Could there really be any truth to storm systems initiating labor?" It certainly seems that way sometimes.

Actually both of my patients really were in labor and I was able to deliver them rather quickly and get a couple hours of sledding in with the kids later that day. The next day I began my investigation into this interesting question. Between 1978 and 1985, there were four studies all of which showed a relationship between dropping barometric pressure and an increase in ruptured membranes. This drop in barometric or atmospheric pressure usually accompanies major storm systems. Since labor usually starts when the amniotic membranes are ruptured, it appears that there is some truth to this common belief.

Even though this fall in pressure seems to bring on an increase in laboring women because of ruptured membranes, it does not appear to bring on labor itself. This was the conclusion from a study from the University of Massachusetts in 1996 involving over two thousand women. When the onset of labor was correlated with the barometric pressure, they found no relationship between the two. So for some reason, membranes seem to be sensitive to pressure changes while the uterus itself is not.

REFERENCES

Boland N, Byers R, Kitay D. *Meteorologic phenomena and labor initiation.* Department of Gynecology and Obstetrics, Emory University School of Medicine 168: Bulletin No. 2, 1980.

Milingos S, Messinis I, Diakomanolis D, Aravantinos D, Kaskarelis D. Influence of meteorological factors on premature rupture of fetal membranes. *Lancet* 2:435, 1978.

Noller KL, Resseguie LJ, and Voss V. The effect of changes in atmospheric pressure on the occurrence of the spontaneous onset of labor in term pregnancies. *Am J Obstet Gynecol* Apr; 174(4): 1192–9, 1996.

Polansky GH, Varner MW, O'Gormn T. Premature rupture of the membranes and barometric pressure changes. *J Reprod Med* 30: 189–91, 1985.

Steinman G, Kleiner G. Spontaneous premature rupture of membranes: correlation with ambient atmospheric pressure. *NY State J Med* 78: 900–1, 1978.

QUESTION: How can you accurately determine when a woman will go into labor?

A. By her last menstrual period.
B. By an ultrasound.
C. By thumping the uterus and hearing a resonant sound much like a ripe melon.
D. None of the above.

ANSWER: D.

A woman's due date is only an estimate of when she will deliver and can never be "accurately" determined. We use a number of criteria to get in the ballpark of when most women will deliver, but none of these criteria can be considered gospel.

The first thing that is used is a woman's last menstrual period. If you take the first day of a woman's last menstrual period, subtract three months, and then add one week, this will give you her due date. This method (which is known as Naegele's rule) makes a few assumptions. First, it assumes that a woman knows the first day of her last menstrual period. When women are not really planning to get pregnant (which includes about half of all couples) or for those who tend to be irregular, they may have no idea when their last period started. For these women, guessing at their last menstrual period can be pretty inaccurate. Secondly, this method assumes that all women have a perfect 28-day cycle and ovulate on day 14. *(If you find this woman, send her to my office because I would like to clone her.)* Most women vary somewhat from this ideal woman, which adds error to the calculation. Thirdly, women can bleed early in pregnancy as the fertilized egg implants into the uterus, and they might incorrectly assume that this was their last menstrual period even though they were already pregnant. It is also possible for a woman to not ovulate the month before she gets pregnant and this will throw the due date calculation off by a month the other way. Lastly, this method assumes that all pregnancies last exactly 40 weeks which just simply isn't true. Anyway, if you take all of the above error into account, this method can still be useful in calculating due dates if a woman has a reasonable idea of when her last menstrual period was and has fairly regular cycles. This calculation will be accurate for most of these women with an error of plus or minus two weeks.

Another way of calculating a due date is to do an ultrasound. As a general rule, the earlier the ultrasound, the more accurate the due date. First trimester calculations have an accuracy of about plus or minus one week, whereas third trimester dates have an error of about plus or minus three weeks. (You can probably look at a pregnant woman's abdomen from across the room in the third trimester and be more accurate than an ultrasound). So it is pretty easily seen that although first trimester ultrasounds are helpful in figuring out due dates, late ultrasounds are fairly worthless for this purpose.

The size of the uterus on the initial prenatal visit can be used to estimate the time of delivery. Some physicians feel they can accurately determine how far along a woman is in the first or early second trimester by feeling the uterus on pelvic exam. I am certainly not one of them. I have been off by as much as three or four weeks at times and use this as one of my least accurate ways of dating a pregnancy.

Quickening refers to when a woman first feels the baby move and has been used in the past to estimate due dates. The average time a woman feels movement is around 20 weeks, but there is a great deal of variation from this. Generally, women who have had previous pregnancies feel movement earlier than those who are first time moms. It is not unusual for women with previous pregnancies to feel movement at 16 or 17 weeks, whereas the newly initiated don't start feeling movement until 22 or 23 weeks. This large difference among women tends to make this method of calculating due dates fairly unreliable.

Fundal height measurement is another technique used by most physicians to continually monitor whether your due date calculations are correct or not. This involves measuring the distance from the pubic bone of a woman to the top of her uterus. The number of centimeters that you get should match how far along the pregnancy is in weeks. For example, if a woman comes in for a prenatal visit at 28 weeks, this measurement should be 28 centimeters. If the measurement is 25 centimeters, then either the baby isn't growing properly or your established due date may be off. An ultrasound may then be ordered to aid in explaining this discrepancy.

As you can see, there is no one way to accurately determine when a woman will actually deliver. A number of criteria, however, may be used to get an idea of approximately when the baby should make its appearance. Generally, if you have a last menstrual period due date for a woman with a reasonable memory and fairly regular periods, along with an early ultrasound that agrees with this date within a couple of weeks, you can estimate the date of arrival within plus or minus two weeks. Realistically, though, we should probably use the words "due range" rather than "due date."

QUESTION: Are first babies usually born late (after the due date)?

A. Absolutely. Especially if it's the middle of August, your air conditioning has gone out, and you feel like Mount Saint Helens right before it erupted.
B. Only if your mother-in-law is planning to stay at your house until junior gets here.
C. Not if your obstetrician (or family practitioner or midwife) is going on vacation when you're due.
D. No. It doesn't matter if it is your first or your tenth—the delivery date has nothing to do with birth order.

ANSWER: D.

As we discussed in previous questions, a pregnancy lasts an average of 280 days or 40 weeks beginning on the first day of a woman's last menstrual period. Due dates are calculated on this average length of pregnancy. It assumes that a woman ovulates around day 14 and has a menstrual cycle length of 28 days. In reality, women's cycles vary greatly and this variation accounts for most of the error in calculating a due date.

In order to take into account this variation in cycle length, a baby is considered "full term" if it is born between 38 and 42 weeks from the first day of the last menstrual period. Before 38 weeks the infant is preterm and after 42 weeks he or she is post-term. This variation in cycle length has nothing to do with the number of pregnancies that a woman has had. I suspect that the misconception of first babies coming late stems from the observation that families eagerly anticipate the birth of their first child. When these couples reach the time around their due date, each day can seem like forever. When this couple actually goes past their due date, the agony of waiting is very memorable. Once you have a child or two, you have less time to concentrate on your pregnancy and time seems to pass much faster. If you do go past your due date, these days are easily forgotten in the hectic turmoil of everyday life.

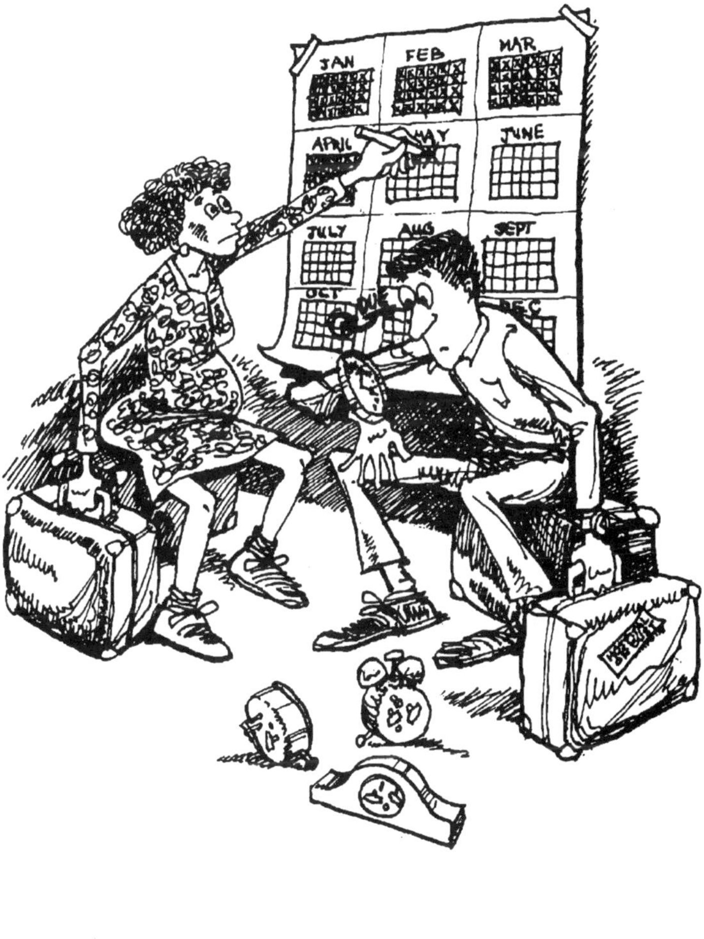

Also remember that actual due dates are based on many factors besides the menstrual age that I have discussed. Some women have extremely irregular cycles or have no recollection of their last menstrual periods. In these cases, ultrasound dating may be used to calculate a due date. Always keep in mind that due dates are approximations and should never be relied upon as exact dates of delivery. In any event, whether a pregnancy is a woman's first or her tenth, she is no more likely to go "early" or "late."

QUESTION: Is labor longer for women delivering for the first time compared to women who have had babies before?

A. Yes.
B. No.
C. It depends if epidurals are used.
D. It depends if you happen to hit your OB's golf day.

ANSWER: A.

In a study by Dr. Friedman in 1978 involving several thousand women, labor patterns were analyzed for first time moms (primiparas) and women with previous children (multiparas). In the multiparous group were women who had at least one other child by a vaginal delivery—Cesarean sections didn't count. All of the women in the study had normal labors resulting in normal vaginal deliveries. The total length of labor for primiparas was about 12 hours (±10 hours), compared to 7 to 8 hrs. (±7 hours) in multiparas. Notice that even though there is a substantial difference in the length of labor, these are averages and there is a lot of variation. So even though the average labor length for first time moms was 12 hours, this varied from 2 to 22 with the average being 12. Likewise there is a ±7 hour variation for multiparas. This difference in labor length based on previous children delivered has been shown by a number of investigators since that time. It is my clinical experience as well as that of most other deliverers of babies that the more children a woman has, the shorter the overall length of labor.

If all of the previous information is true, why then was grandma in labor for three weeks with all five of her children whereas Aunt Susie delivered her first in her husband's pickup truck on Interstate 75 on the way to the hospital. *(By the way Uncle Frank did manage to toss her in the flat bed in back moments before her water broke thereby sparing his new Corinthian leather. Unfortunately the flat bed was filled with freshly picked roses from their garden. The baby was fine, but to this day, Aunt Susie is finding thorns in her backside. You might also say that Uncle Frank's life has not been a bed of roses since that memorable delivery.)* Getting back to the point, many women have uncomfortable uterine activity hours, days, or even weeks before labor actually hits. Other women seem to have an unusually high tolerance for pain. They can be quite far along in labor before becoming uncomfortable and labor can progress rapidly. Therefore pain tolerance is an important factor along with birth order.

So for the most part, you first time moms can hang around the house a little longer when labor starts, but some of you multips might need to head out earlier—but don't forget about variations in pain tolerance. As far as you fathers-to-be go, hold off on the new car until after the baby gets here.

REFERENCES

Creasy RK, Resnik R. *Maternal Fetal Medicine.* Third edition. W.B. Saunders Co. Phila., Pa. pp. 527–29, 1994.

Friedman EA. Labor: *Clinical Evaluation and Management.* Second edition. Appleton-Century-Crofts. New York, N.Y., 1978.

QUESTION: Can you predict when a woman will deliver by doing a cervical exam in the office?

A. Yes. The more dilated you are, the sooner you will deliver.
B. Yes. The more dilated you are, the later that you will deliver.
C. No. Cervical dilation has nothing to do with when you will deliver. It serves as a baseline for future reference and to more accurately determine fetal position.
D. No. Cervical examinations were invented by male physicians just to make your life a little more miserable as you approach your delivery date.

ANSWER: C.

For some women, cervical exams are one of the most hated parts of going to their prenatal visits. Depending on the examiner and the situation, they can be no big deal, a bit uncomfortable, or down right miserable. Just what information can your physician or midwife get out of this exam and are they really necessary?

First of all, cervical exams are usually performed with a patient lying on her back with her legs positioned in stirrups. The examiner places a gloved, lubricated finger or two into the vagina and locates the cervix (or opening of the uterus) in the back of the vagina. He or she then tries to tell if the cervix is closed or beginning to open. An estimate is then made as to how thick the cervix is (or its effacement) and how far dilated it is.

You can get a pretty good mental picture of how the cervix operates by picturing the uterus as a big, muscular balloon. The part of the balloon that you blow up, we will call the cervix. The baby lives inside this balloon and the opening of the balloon (the cervix) can be found in the back of the vagina. During labor, the large, round muscular part of the uterus contracts around the baby and forces the baby downward. The baby's head presses on the cervix as it moves down and forces it to open up. *(Is there any wonder why the little tykes head resembles a banana squash at delivery after being used as a battering ram during labor?)* As the head presses on the cervix, it first thins out (or effaces), and then begins to give way (or dilate) as the head passes through it and into the vagina. Therefore in labor, we can check a woman's cervix and see how well the baby is moving downward. You see, even though we talk about the cervix effacing and dilating, it really doesn't do anything. It just gives way as the big, muscular uterus contracts down and forces the baby out. Most women start labor with their cervix either not dilated at all, or possibly dilated up to a few centimeters. When the head has come all the way through, the cervix is paper thin and dilated to about ten centimeters. We call this being completely dilated, and at this time a woman is ready to start the second stage of labor, which is pushing the baby out.

Now that you understand the function of the cervix in labor, let's get back to the original question. Why do you need to check a woman's cervix in the office before she starts labor? Actually, there is not total agreement among physicians concerning this question. Some physicians believe that you can predict who will go into labor prematurely by checking the cervix. They therefore check a woman's cervix on each visit and if they are starting to dilate or efface prematurely, they will place a woman at bed rest or possibly start medications to prevent preterm labor. Other physicians (including myself) don't subscribe to this theory and only check a woman's cervix if she begins having regular contractions and appears to be in labor. An exception to this would be if a woman has a history of an incompetent cervix. These women have usually lost a pregnancy in the past because the cervix is weak and dilates completely just from the weight of the baby. These women need to be watched very closely and may even need to have a stitch placed in their cervix to keep it from dilating prematurely.

Somewhere in the last month of pregnancy, virtually all physicians begin to check the cervix for two main reasons. First of all, you can more accurately determine a baby's position vaginally than abdominally. Vaginally it is possible to feel the firmness and roundness of the baby's head and establish that it is in the correct position. If a baby is breech (rear end first) or transverse (sideways), it is fairly easy to feel this (by feeling a much softer, squishier butt or getting kicked by a foot) and then know that the baby is not in the desired position. The optimum time to find out that a baby is not head first is about 37 weeks. At this time, the physician may decide to try to turn the baby around into the correct position by pressing on a woman's abdomen using a technique called external version. *(By the way, don't try this at home. Besides making the baby a bit dizzy, this technique can do some weird things to the umbilical cord and get the little varmint decidedly upset. External versions should be done in labor and delivery under ultrasound guidance).* Thirty-seven weeks is the best time to do this because if you try it earlier, the baby is small enough and there is enough fluid around the baby to allow it to turn back to the wrong position. If you try this maneuver much later than 37 weeks, the baby is usually too big, and there is not an adequate amount of fluid to allow it to be done successfully.

The second reason to do a cervical exam in the last month of pregnancy is to get a baseline for that patient's cervix. If a woman has a dilation, for instance, of one centimeter in the office and then later that night calls you thinking that she is in labor, this information may be helpful. When she comes in to labor and delivery, you can check her cervix and see if it is beginning to dilate. If she is still one centimeter, then the contractions aren't strong enough to move the baby downward to change the cervix and you can determine that she is in false labor. If she is three centimeters, then she is most likely in labor. So the office cervical examine can serve as a baseline for future reference, BUT IT CAN'T PREDICT WHEN A WOMAN WILL GO INTO LABOR! Let me clarify this a bit. Whether a woman's cervix is long and closed in the office or is four centimeters dilated, it doesn't make her any more likely to go into labor. As a general rule, the more children a woman has had, the more likely she is to be a little more dilated when she starts labor. We currently have a patient in our practice that is five centimeters dilated with her fifth child but is not in labor. So don't be disappointed when your doc tells you that your cervix is long and closed on your office exam. You are just as likely to go into labor as the patient that is dilated three or four centimeters.

Myths & Facts of Risk

From the moment a woman finds out she is pregnant, she is surrounded by what Vicki Iovine in her book *The Girlfriends' Guide to Pregnancy* calls the Pregnancy Police. *(By the way, her book is a real hoot and is definitely worth reading).* You know who I mean. All of those "well-meaning" friends and relatives who love to tell you about how your baby will resemble Godzilla because you drink tap water instead of the chic new bottled variety or that the glass of wine you had in your first trimester will keep your kid from entering Harvard. *(Coincidentally, these are also the women who were in labor for four weeks, were given nails to chew on instead of anesthesia, and returned to work on a road crew three days after their delivery).* This segment is the longest as there are quite a few RISK questions out there. Hopefully this chapter will give you some ammunition to use against the dreaded Pregnancy Police.

QUESTION: Can hot tubs cause birth defects?

A. Only if the bubbles are kept on high for long periods of time.
B. Possibly if a pregnant woman is exposed to high temperatures for a long time, but the risk is pretty small.
C. Depends what activities are occurring in the tub.
D. Only in California.

ANSWER: B.

What a bummer! You've spent a whole year planning a second honeymoon to the Poconos. The kids will be at Grandma's for the week. You have worked overtime to be able to get a week off from work and then *BAM*—three days before you leave, "the rabbit dies." Of course you're happy that number three is on the way, but you had the deluxe suite with a heart-shaped hot tub picked out and had visions of a bubbly rendezvous in the moonlight in between sips of champagne. You know that the champagne is off limits, but do you really have to give up that heart-shaped hot tub? Well, let's look at the evidence.

Two studies in the 1970s suggested that exposing pregnant women to increased levels of heat during pregnancy led to increased birth defects. The heat could come from sources such as hot tubs, sunbathing, or prolonged high fevers. These studies were retrospective meaning that they talked to women after delivery and asked them about their exposure to heat during their pregnancy. The obvious flaw with these studies is that they relied on women's memories many months down the line. As any woman with a newborn will tell you, remembering what you did yesterday is a feat, let alone what you did last year.

In 1992, Milunsky followed 5,566 women in New England throughout their pregnancies and noted their exposure to hot tubs, saunas, fever, and electric blankets. He found that if a woman used a hot tub early in pregnancy, she had almost a three times greater risk of having a child with a neural tube (brain or spinal cord) defect than women who didn't use hot tubs. The risk for saunas and fevers was almost twice normal, and there was no increased risk for women using electric blankets.

When the normal risk of a child having a neural tube defect such as spina bifida is 1 to 2 per 1000 deliveries, your risk of having a child with this problem is still small even if you are involved with one of the above activities. None the less, it seems reasonable to stay away from hot tubs and saunas as much as possible during early pregnancy (4 to 14 weeks) when the neural tube is being formed. In regard to hot tubs specifically, it is only the heat of the water that poses any potential harm. Therefore, my advice is to cool down the water and have a blast.

REFERENCES

Creasy RK, Resnick R. *Maternal Fetal Medicine.* W B Saunders Co. Phila., Pa. Third edition. p. 179, 1994.

Milunsky A, Ulcickas M, Rothman KJ, et al. Maternal heat exposure and neural tube defects. *JAMA* 268: 882, 1992.

QUESTION: Can emotional stress adversely affect a pregnancy?

A. Yes. There is evidence that stress may play a role in premature deliveries which in turn leads to smaller birth weight babies.
B. Yes. Stress may lead to an increased chance of miscarriage but has little effect later in pregnancy.
C. Absolutely not. There has never been any evidence that stress effects pregnancy one way or the other. That's only grandma talking.
D. Stress...What's that? The technological explosion that has occurred in our culture has virtually eliminated stress as a factor in our lives.

ANSWER: A.

Boy did this question open a can of worms. In going back over ten years I found no less than 140 studies that addressed this subject. One of the problems inherent in evaluating this statement is that women frequently have an increased amount of stress in their lives from other factors which may affect their pregnancies. For instance, stress-free women eat better and smoke less than stressed-out women. You therefore need to consider the effect of these health factors when evaluating the impact of stress. Moreover, how do you evaluate stress levels in women? For the women of war-torn countries, stress may involve trying to stay alive from day to day whereas for the women of "middle America," it may mean the loss of a job or close family member. Nonetheless, I have waded through all of the literature and will attempt to make some sense of it all.

A common theme which comes up in many studies is that emotional stress seems to be related to an increase in premature deliveries and a decrease in infant birth weight. In the late 1980s, Williamson, et. al. at the University of Missouri studied 513 women from four rural communities. Life stress scores were calculated for these women at various times throughout their pregnancies. The women were then divided into two groups. One group had an overall increase in stress from the second to the third trimester, and the second group had no increase in their stress levels. The group that experienced the increase in stress had a 9.2 percent incidence of a poor outcome in their pregnancy, whereas the non-stressed group had a 3.9 percent incidence. Poor outcome was defined as low birth weight, increased intensive care unit time, and infant death. Since that time, numerous other studies have been done. The majority of studies seem to imply that stress plays a role in fetal outcome, but others question its impact. As I previously stated, it is difficult to completely control for other risk factors such as diet, prenatal care, access to health care, socioeconomic status, smoking, and drug use. These might account for the variations in the results of some of these studies.

One way to correct for some of the above variables is to perform experiments with our friends the rats. Rats, you see, are generally pretty easy folks to study. You can control where they live, what they eat and drink, and how much they smoke. They also don't complain much and love trying to get pregnant. In the late 1980s, Rojo-Fernandez, et. al. and Weller, et. al. took pregnant rats and created stress in their lives by restraining them at various times during their pregnancy. Just for the record, there is one thing that pregnant female rats really hate and that's being tied down. It interferes with their shopping excursions to the mall, hair appointments, jazzercize classes, and has the general effect of making them just plain mean. When these stressed rats gave birth, their offspring were compared to the offspring of non-stressed rats. Lo and behold, the researchers found that the offspring of the stressed rats showed a decreased ability to learn and had a higher overall death rate. These results are consistent with some human research which shows higher rates of attention deficit disorder and general psychological problems in the children of women who have had high levels of stress during their pregnancies.

If stress has the ability to affect pregnancy negatively, what can we do to keep this effect to a minimum? Whether you are a health care provider for a pregnant woman or her friend or relative, support at times of stress can mean a great deal to her. This concept of reducing stress was studied by a group in New Zealand. They studied women who were either single or in a relationship where their partner was unemployed. In other words, they selected a group of women who were at high risk for stressful events. Half were given weekly telephone calls by caring health care providers and half were not. The telephone support group had less overall anxiety and depression as well as higher self-esteem. So even a simple weekly telephone call may make a big difference in a woman's anxiety level and potentially affect the outcome of her pregnancy.

In summary, there are many conflicting studies concerning stress as it relates to pregnancy outcome. Stress does not appear to have a relationship to early pregnancy loss, but can play a role in premature deliveries resulting in babies of decreased birth weight and development. It is our job as health care providers, friends, and family members to help decrease this stress in any way we can.

REFERENCES

Bullock LF, Wells JE, Duff GB, Hornblow AR. Telephone support for pregnant women: outcome in late pregnancy. *N Z Med J* Nov 24; 108(1012): 476–8, 1995.

McIntosh DE, Mulkins RS, Dean RA. Utilization of maternal perinatal risk indicators in the differential diagnosis of ADHD and UADD children. *Int J Neurosci* Mar; 81(1–2): 35–46, 1995.

Rojo-Fernandez M, Marin B, Menendez-Patterson A. Effects of immobilization stress in utero of the course of pregnancy in the rat and on various parameters in the newborn animals. *Rev Esp Fisiol* Mar; 41(1): 29–35, 1985.

Ward AJ. Prenatal stress and childhood psychopathology. *Child Psychiatry Hum Dev* Winter: 22(2): 97–110, 1991.

Weller A, Glaubman H, Yehuda S, Caspy T, Ben-Uria Y. Acute and repeated gestational stress affect offspring learning and activity in rats. *Physiol Behav* 43;(2): 139–43,1988.

Williamson HA, LeFevre M, Hector M. Association between life stress and serious perinatal complications. *J Fam Pract* Nov: 29(5): 489–96, 1989.

QUESTION: Is radiation exposure (such as from x-rays) harmful during pregnancy?

A. Yes…in any dose anytime in pregnancy.
B. Yes…in high doses late in pregnancy.
C. Yes…in high doses early in pregnancy.
D. No. Radiation has no effect on pregnancy.

ANSWER: C.

If you've said it once, you've said it a thousand times—"Put your toys away when you're finished playing." Sure enough, though, you get up early one morning and go to the kitchen to get breakfast started and *KABOOM!*—down you go after tripping on a studmobile complete with Barbie and Ken. You land right on your tush and an electric shock starts at your tailbone and exits through your eye teeth. "This is it," you say to yourself, "I've definitely broken something now." You crawl back into the bedroom and shake your husband awake. After explaining your morning escapade, he helps you and the kids into the car and you are off to the emergency room.

Fortunately the pelvic x-rays are negative and you leave the hospital with an inflatable doughnut and a mild case of embarrassment at having your derriere scrutinized by an intern, nurse, chief resident, and a radiology technician. All agreed that nothing was broken and nominated you for the "I can't sit down for a month" club. Just as you arrive home, one of their questions comes to mind and you break out in a cold sweat. "Could you be pregnant?" they had asked. "Of course not," you told them. It's true that your period is two weeks late, but your cycles are always irregular and the two of you are very careful (whatever that means). Just to ease your mind, however, your husband runs to the store and buys the Acme Do It Yourself Home Pregnancy Test. After reading the "easy" directions, you spend the next half hour trying to pee in a cup that you can barely see. *(Surely these tests were devised by guys with a great sense of humor.)* You mix the appropriate solutions and *BINGO*...another bun in the oven! Your emotions go from surprise to acceptance to panic when you think back to the x-rays you received earlier that morning. You could kick yourself for not suspecting the pregnancy and are pretty scared that you might have already harmed your new addition. The next call is usually to your obstetrician/midwife to inquire about the risk to the baby.

There is no doubt that at certain doses, radiation is harmful to a fetus—but what exactly are those doses and when should you worry that your baby may have been harmed. Doses of radiation that are less than 5 rads (rads are just a way of measuring radiation exposure) are known to be safe for a baby in the first trimester. The first trimester is when all of the organs are forming and when a baby is most sensitive to radiation. Doses greater than 10 rads have been known to cause birth defects. Between 5 and 10 rads is a zone of relative uncertainty. The amount of radiation that you were exposed to by the x-rays this morning was 41 millirads or 41 one thousandths of 1 rad—an astronomically small amount of radiation. In fact, most of the common x-rays that are done today expose you to much less than 1 rad. This is not to say that you should ignore the risks of radiation exposure during pregnancy, but simply put it in perspective if it unknowingly happens. So in this case, you can sit back (on your doughnut) and prepare yourself for the first trimester barfing that is about to start and know that your new little one will probably not glow in the dark.

REFERENCES

Creasy RK, Resnick R. *Maternal Fetal Medicine.* WB Saunders Co. Phila., Pa. Third edition. p.178, 1994.

Swartz HM, Reichling BA. Hazards of radiation exposure for pregnant women. *JAMA* 239: 1907. 1978.

QUESTION: Can eating too much salt or gaining too much weight during pregnancy cause a woman to develop toxemia?

A. Yes. Studies have proven that there is a link between salt consumption, weight gain, and toxemia.
B. Studies haven't proven this relationship, but they certainly suggest a possible connection.
C. Eating salt and gaining weight can actually prevent toxemia.
D. No. Salt consumption and weight gain have nothing to do with the development of toxemia.

ANSWER: D.

Toxemia refers to a condition that affects about 7 percent of all pregnant women. Classically, these women develop high blood pressure, protein in their urine, and swelling within the third trimester (the last three months) of their pregnancy. It tends to affect women at the extremes of the age range, both teenagers and more mature women *(just trying to be politically correct)* and also tends to affect first pregnancies more often than future ones. Although there are a number of theories that address why some women develop this condition and others do not, the true cause is unknown.

The term toxemia dates back to many years ago when it was thought that these women had a poison or toxin in their blood that was responsible for the development of this affliction. Today we know there is no specific toxin responsible for the problem, and we use the terms pregnancy-induced hypertension or preeclampsia when referring to this condition. Since pregnancy-induced hypertension also includes other hypertensive problems of pregnancy, I will use the more specific term, preeclampsia.

Preeclampsia occurs when many of the blood vessels around the body go into a sort of spasm during pregnancy, which accounts for the rise in blood pressure. This total body vascular spasm leads to decreased blood flow to many organs in the body including the kidneys, placenta, and the brain. When the kidneys don't get enough blood, they aren't able to do their job which is to filter out the "bad stuff" in the blood and keep the "good stuff." The good stuff is a variety of proteins, and when the kidneys are unable to hang on to these proteins, they escape into the urine. Therefore this protein in the urine may be a sign of decreased kidney function. If blood vessels spasm in the placenta, there is decreased blood flow to the baby and the baby may have stunted growth or even die. If left unchecked, these vessels may also spasm in the mother's brain leading to strokes or seizures. (When a woman seizes, she is then said to have eclampsia). To this day, there is no real treatment for this condition except to deliver the baby. If preeclampsia is picked up early and delivery is carried out, most moms and babies do well provided that the baby is far enough along.

Why then, is there this mistaken notion that salt restriction or diet modification will prevent preeclampsia? The salt restriction concept relates to hypertension that develops in non-pregnant adults over time. This type of hypertension is called essential hypertension and seems to get worse in people who have high salt diets. Since salt affects this type of hypertension, many people assume that it might also lead to hypertension in pregnancy. Quite simply, it does not.

In regard to weight gain causing preeclampsia, the story goes like this. In preeclamptic women, vascular spasm occurs, which forces fluid out of the blood vessels and into the surrounding tissues. This accounts for the swelling that is seen. As the condition progresses, more and more fluid is forced into the tissue spaces, which increases swelling and overall weight gain due to water retention. So in reality, the weight gain is a result of the preeclampsia, but does not cause it. Something else I hear rather often is the concept that if you eat a high protein diet, you can avoid preeclampsia. This comes from the thought that if you return to the body the protein that it is losing in the urine, preeclampsia may be avoided. Ixnay to this idea too.

Fortunately today we can usually avoid complications of preeclampsia with good prenatal care. This involves taking a pregnant woman's blood pressure and checking for urine protein each visit, along with recognizing the symptoms of preeclampsia. These symptoms can include headache, blurred vision, seeing spots, and pain in the upper abdomen. If this condition is recognized early and delivery is carried out, serious consequences can usually be avoided.

So you can stock up on those three Ps of pure pleasure with a clear conscience as far as preeclampsia is concerned—pretzels, potato chips, and pastries. What it does to your waistline is another question.

REFERENCES

Creasy RK, Resnick R. *Maternal Fetal Medicine.* Third edition. W.B. Saunders Co. Philadelphia, Pa. 806–838, 1994.

Cunningham FG, MacDonald PC, Gant NF, Leveno KJ, Gilstrap LC. *Williams Obstetrics.* 19th edition. Appleton & Lange. Norwalk, Conn. pp. 763–803, 1993.

QUESTION: Are hair dyes and perm agents dangerous to use during pregnancy?

A. Yes. They are extremely dangerous anytime in pregnancy.
B. Yes. They are dangerous but only in the first trimester in any dose and not nearly as dangerous as the grey, straight, and stringy "witch look" you'll get from not using them.
C. Yes, but only in the first trimester when large doses are used.
D. There is little evidence to support the idea that these chemicals cause any harm during the entire pregnancy at any dose.

ANSWER: D.

You can pretty well throw this one into the myth category. My literature search came up with plenty of rat studies that tried to address the issue of hair dyes and birth defects. Why rats? Well, it's fairly hard to convince pregnant women today to take part in a study of this variety. Our furry friends seem to be the lucky winners. When these little critters are exposed to whopping doses of chemicals that are commonly used by today's hairdressers, there don't seem to be any negative effects on their kids. In fact, they have been reported to be seen strutting around town with their litter of newborns all sporting their new "do's." I am told that the latest new style is the *cheese curl.*

The best source of human information that we have is a literature search by a Scandinavian group that looked at reproductive disorders of hairdressers from 1985 through 1993. Since this segment of the population is continually exposed to numerous hair chemicals, this is as close as we can get to human studies on these agents. Their conclusion was that there is little evidence for reproductive disorders in this group. It would seem from the above animal studies and this literature review that commonly used hair preparations are relatively safe in pregnancy. Many of the hairdressers I interviewed agreed with this statement. They were quick to add, however, that perms are probably not a good idea in pregnancy as they lose their curl very rapidly yielding an unhappy customer. An informal discussion with my rat friends around town also verified this coiffural fact of life.

REFERENCES

DiNardo JC, Picciano JC, Schnetzinger RW, Morris WE, Wolf BA: Teratological assessment of five oxidative hair dyes in the rat. *Toxicol Appl Pharmacol* Mar 30; 78(1): 163–6, 1985.

Kersemaekers WM, Roeleveld N, Zielhuis GA: Reproductive disorders due to chemical exposure among hairdressers. *Scand J Work Environ Health* Oct; 21(5): 325–34, 1995.

QUESTION: Does eating candy and other sweets during pregnancy cause you to develop diabetes?

A. Definitely not. Aren't Baby Ruth bars one of the main food groups?
B. Eating sweets doesn't cause you to develop diabetes, but can make it worse for those who do develop it.
C. There is absolutely no relationship between sugar and diabetes.
D. Only women who are diabetics before they become pregnant have to worry about eating sweets.

ANSWER: B.

Diabetes mellitus occurs in 1 to 3 percent of all pregnancies making it one of the most common complications of pregnancy. Prior to the discovery of insulin in 1921, most diabetics were too ill to become pregnant. Of those that did, 25 percent of the mothers and 50 percent of the infants died. With the use of insulin today, the maternal and fetal mortality is close to that of non-diabetic patients. Today, we generally divide pregnant diabetics into two groups: 1) overt diabetics who have their disease prior to becoming pregnant and 2) gestational diabetics who develop their problem sometime during pregnancy. The question here really is, "Does what you eat lead to developing gestational diabetes?"

To fully answer the above question, let me regress for a minute and go over some basic concepts about gestational diabetes. Everything you eat is broken down in the stomach and small intestine into simple sugars that are transported in the bloodstream to all of the cells of the body. These cells then use the sugar as an energy source so that you can do things like read this book or practice conceiving that next child *(if you are skillful, maybe even at the same time).* In order to get the sugar from the bloodstream into the cells, the body needs a hormone called insulin. Insulin, which is produced by the pancreas, needs to be in adequate supply to ensure that the sugar is able to get from the bloodstream into the cells. Most of us have excellent insulin reserves to cover for things like the three pieces of sugar cream pie you snarfed down last night. If you don't have enough insulin around, however, then the sugar remains in the bloodstream and doesn't get into the cells. This makes the level of sugar in the bloodstream very high, and in a pregnant woman these high levels of sugar can easily cross through the placenta and into the baby's bloodstream. The baby takes one look at all these yummy snack cakes headed its way, looks toward the heavens, and says, "Thank you, Lord." Unlike mama, the baby has adequate levels of insulin and can easily transport this sugar into its own cells giving him or her the appearance of the Michelin Tire Man if this process is not halted. It must be like working in a Hershey's factory as a candy sampler.

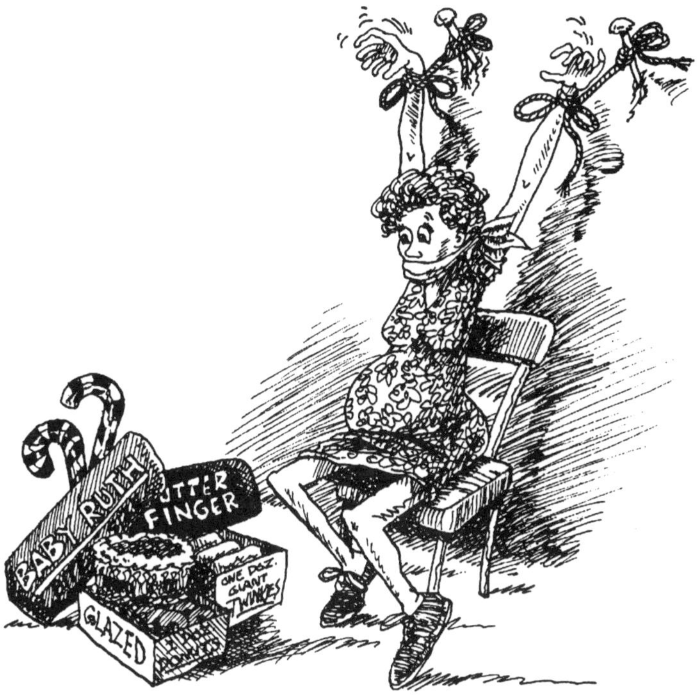

Although junior is rather thrilled at this tasty development, there are a couple of negative effects of this newfound "mother lode" that make us want to stem the tide. First of all, when these kids develop their sumo wrestler–like body appearance, it can make for difficult deliveries and increase the need for Cesarean sections. Second of all, remember that at delivery, the cord is clamped, which puts a drastic halt to the little kiddo's pipeline of Baby Ruth bars. The baby's insulin levels before delivery are at all-time highs, so when the caravan of sugar is halted, the baby's sugar levels plummet. Obviously, this can make for a less than happy youngster as intravenous sugars are needed to stabilize the baby at birth. Eventually, the baby's insulin and sugar levels balance out appropriately, but this may take place over a number of days and lead to a great deal of anxiety within the parents.

To directly answer this question, some women naturally have less insulin reserves than others, and that is why some women develop diabetes in pregnancy. Pregnant women today are tested for diabetes between 24 and 28 weeks by giving them a sugary solution to drink down and then drawing their blood one hour later to see how they can handle the sugar. If it is determined that they have gestational diabetes, their diet may be manipulated to decrease the amount of simple sugars they eat. These women are then monitored by checking their blood sugars throughout pregnancy. If simple diet manipulation does not keep their blood sugars in line, they must give themselves insulin. So even though you can't "make yourself" become diabetic during pregnancy, diet plays a big role in the treatment of gestational diabetes.

REFERENCES

Cunningham FG, MacDonald, MD, Gant NF, Leveno, KJ, Gilstrap LC. *Williams Obstetrics.* 19th edition. Appleton & Lange. Norwalk, Conn. pp. 1201–12, 1993.

QUESTION: Can lying flat on your back during pregnancy can injure the baby?

A. Yes, but only after several hours.
B. Yes, even brief periods of time on your back can injure the baby.
C. Theoretically yes, but your body has built in safeguards that won't allow this to happen.
D. No. Babies are equally happy whether you are on your back, side, or abdomen.

ANSWER: C.

Open just about any book related to pregnancy and somewhere between the covers you will invariably find a passage that warns about the dangers of lying flat on your back during pregnancy. Is this really detrimental to the little guy (or girl), or do these authors simply enjoy printing frightening material. The answer to this question is that there is an element of truth to this statement, but it needs to be put in its proper perspective. Allow me to explain.

First of all I need to give you a brief and painless anatomy lesson. *(Calm down...I said it would be brief).* The uterus is a muscle that resides in the center of the pelvis. As it becomes larger throughout pregnancy, it eventually occupies the entire lower abdomen. As it so happens, the uterus lies directly over top of a large vein called the vena cava *(Stick with me here. I promise that it will get a little more interesting).* This vena cava brings all of the oxygen-poor blood from the lower half of the body back to the heart and lungs to be reoxygenated and pumped out again to the rest of the body. As the uterus gets bigger, it puts pressure on the vena cava, which tends to impede blood flow back to the heart and keep blood pooled in the legs. That's why pregnant women tend to have a great deal of swelling in their legs as pregnancy progresses. If a pregnant woman lies directly on her back, the uterus squashes the vena cava against the backbone and causes maximum compression. When this occurs, there is less blood available to be pumped out to important things like the placenta, which makes junior a little perturbed. This is the basis for saying that lying on your back is harmful to the baby.

If a pregnant woman continues to remain in this position, can it really cause some kind of damage to the baby? Well...theoretically yes, but practically, this is a lot of bunk. I like to draw parallels to this concept of hurting the baby by lying on your back and a bratty little kid I knew once. One day, he informed his parents that he was royally upset with them and would hold his breath until he died. *(What better way to get to your parents than a little threatened death?).* The wise parents simply provided an ample amount of pillows around me...I mean the little kid...and after he held his breath for as long as he could, he briefly fainted, started breathing normally, and gazed into the faces of his smiling parents. The moral of this story has nothing to do with triumph of parental wisdom over a child's temper tantrum, but is that your body takes pretty good care of you. It generally won't let you harm yourself. This laying on your back issue falls into the same category. If a pregnant woman squashes the vena cava enough to decrease blood flow to the baby, then blood flow is also decreased to important things like the brain. Your brain says something like, *"Roll over on your side stupid, I don't feel so good,"* and you magically roll over on your side thereby promoting better blood flow. In fact, if you ask pregnant women which sleeping position they prefer later in pregnancy, most will tell you it's on their side. If you ask them to pick which side, they will usually say their left side as the vena cava actually runs along the right side of the body, and this position gets the uterus off of the vena cava a little better.

This same principle accounts for pregnant women continually becoming light-headed and sometimes fainting when sitting or standing for long periods of time. Prolonged sitting or standing (like attending a long church service or riding in a car for hours on end) can further contribute to pooling of the blood in the legs, which momentarily may deprive the brain of its share of that all important oxygen. If it is not corrected by changing position, the woman's brain may get a little honked off and make a spectacle of her by forcing her on her side via fainting. This principle is utilized in most labor and delivery units through the country as they continually place laboring women on their sides during labor. This appeases the future new arrival and makes Mom's experience a lot more enjoyable.

In reality, your body takes pretty darn good care of you and won't allow major catastrophes like doing your kid in through positional blunders. So when you find yourself waking up in the middle of the night lying flat on your back, don't worry that you have done some irrevocable harm to the little bambino. Just roll over and drift back off to sleep knowing that your little one is safe and sound.

QUESTION: Does traveling in airplanes during pregnancy cause premature rupture of membranes?

A. Yes. It increases your chances of rupturing membranes approximately ten times.
B. Depends what you're doing on the plane and who you're doing it with.
C. Only with women who have high-risk pregnancies.
D. No. There is no evidence to support this.

ANSWER: D.

This was a toughy. In my literature search back to 1966 on this subject, I found zilch, nada, and zippo. There was one obscure study from the University of Hawaii that looked at 33 tourists who delivered prematurely at their hospital from 1984–89. A total of 37 infants were born to these women *(yes, there were some multiple births...I'm glad that you are paying attention),* and all of them required care in their intensive care unit. When the histories of these women were analyzed, it was found that 30 percent of them had factors that placed them at high risk for delivering prematurely.

A previous study from 1978–84 from the same university saw 27 infants born prematurely during that time period, and 50 percent of these women had high risk factors. Their conclusion was that women with high risk factors for delivering prematurely should not travel long distances. *NO DUH!!!* My personal, creative conclusion differs slightly from theirs. Let me explain. Fifty percent of the women who delivered prematurely in Hawaii from 1978–84 had high risk factors placing them at risk for delivering prematurely. From 1984–1989, however, only 30 percent of the women who delivered prematurely had high risk factors. That means over an 11 year period, the number of women with high risk factors decreased by 20 percent. Therefore, we should send all of our pregnant women on trips to Hawaii and eventually we will eliminate all high risk factors for delivering prematurely. In looking at all of the money this might save by reducing preterm deliveries and neonatal intensive care costs, insurance companies should be mandated to pick up the costs of these therapeutic trips. Furthermore, until the high risk factors are reduced to zero, obstetricians and their families should accompany these patients and their families to ensure good continuity of care.

On a slightly more serious note, there seems to be no data to support the idea that air travel will predispose a pregnant woman to prematurely rupturing her membranes. What I tell most of my non–high-risk patients is that travel is okay any time during their pregnancy, but that as they get close to their due date, it makes sense to stay relatively close to home. This will ensure that when they go into labor, they will be surrounded by familiar medical personnel. For those patients who choose to travel, the only disadvantage they may have is delivering in a strange town with unfamiliar people attending to their care. So most of my patients travel pretty freely during their pregnancy by whatever method of transportation is most convenient. High-risk women usually stay relatively close to home once they reach the time of fetal viability (roughly the third trimester). Even if these women must travel and happen to run into problems, there are very few places at least in this country that can't offer level two or three delivery units within a reasonable distance. So don't let travel scare you during pregnancy and remember to write to your congress person to lobby for prenatal trips to Hawaii complete with obstetrical coverage from yours truly.

REFERENCES

Easa D, Pelke S, Loo SW, Ash K. Unexpected preterm delivery in tourists: implications for long distance travel during pregnancy. *J Perinatol* Jul–Aug: 14(4): 264–7, 1994.

QUESTION: Is it safe to wear a seat belt when you are pregnant?

A. Not only is it safe and highly recommended, but in some states, it's the law.
B. It's safe but the lap belt should be adjusted to rest above the uterus to avoid injuring the baby.
C. No. pressure from the seat belt could be harmful to the baby.
D. They are safe but seat belts have really never been shown to be of benefit for anyone whether they are pregnant or not.

ANSWER: A.

The answer to this question should be pretty obvious. We all know that pregnant women should always wear seat belts, right? Well, evidently not. In a recent study involving a large U.S. military installation, a questionnaire was sent to all of their undelivered pregnant women. This questionnaire asked a number of questions regarding current and past use of seat belts. A full 23 percent of these women were either misinformed or uninformed concerning seat belt usage during pregnancy. Another non-governmental survey done a few years earlier revealed that less than half of the pregnant women interviewed reported using seat belts regularly and almost one third of the women who used seat belts did not adjust them properly. The blame for this misinformation lies not with the public, however, but with health care providers like myself. This was apparent in a third survey involving 236 board-certified obstetrician–gynecologists randomly selected in California. (I can assure you that the results would be similar here in Ohio or in any other state for that matter.) When asked about seat belt safety during pregnancy, one out of four physicians either could not give an opinion or had doubts about the safety of using seat belts in pregnancy. Pretty wild, huh? Moreover, fewer than one third of these physicians discussed maternal or infant/child seat belt safety with their patients at some time during their pregnancy.

What's the big deal anyway? Is car restraint safety really all that important? Does it impact enough of our patients to warrant giving up some of our precious office time to discuss it? Well, let me put it this way. What is the single most common cause of maternal death in this country? Is it bleeding during delivery or ruptured tubal pregnancies? Maybe it's stroke due to hypertension or preeclampsia. How about complications secondary to uncontrolled diabetes. Nope. *THE LARGEST SINGLE CAUSE OF MATERNAL DEATH IN THIS COUNTRY IS FROM TRAUMA DUE TO AUTOMOBILE ACCIDENTS!* Somewhere between three and four hundred pregnant women will die each year in automobile accidents, and what is most important about this fact is that both the fetal and maternal death rates are significantly higher in unrestrained women. As an example, a three-year study from Victoria, Australia showed that there were 5 maternal and 27 fetal deaths due to automobile accidents. Although there were fetal deaths in both restrained and unrestrained women, all maternal deaths were in the unrestrained group. Another U.S. study agreed with the Australian study and showed that unrestrained pregnant women were roughly twice as likely to give birth to a low birth weight baby and to deliver within 48 hours of the accident. Likewise, air bags have been shown to improve maternal survival—especially in head on collisions.

Is there any down side to seat belts or air bags? Very little. We all have heard of reports where there has been a uterine rupture or placental abruption (where the placenta pulls away from the uterus) in a pregnant woman who was wearing a seat belt. Undoubtedly, there will be both fetal and maternal deaths in restrained women, but on the whole, the number and severity of injuries sustained in an accident will be significantly reduced by wearing seat belts. As for air bags, people will certainly sustain minor injuries such as abrasions of the face, neck, chest, and arms as well as chemical irritations from the powder covering the air bag, but fatalities are seen to be drastically reduced when air bags are used. Keep in mind, however, that when air bags are in place in the front seat, children and small adults should be placed in the back seat. Major injuries and fatalities have resulted from the impact of the bags with smaller folks.

When a pregnant patient is involved in an automobile accident, it is extremely important to have her evaluated in the hospital no matter how minor the injuries seem. This recommendation is based on information out of Ontario, Canada. In the years 1982–86, all traumatic fetal deaths were reviewed by the chief coroner's office of Ontario. They found that there were 13 cases reported during this time period. All of the deaths occurred in fetuses who were in the third trimester (last three months of pregnancy). In 8 of these cases, the injuries to the mother were considered minor, and half of these women were actually discharged from the hospital only to be found to have a fetal demise at a later time. Besides finding that the amount of maternal trauma did not always correlate with the amount of fetal damage, they also noted that seat belts were worn in only 4 of the 13 cases. In light of these findings, all pregnant women who have been involved in an accident should be evaluated in the emergency room for any evidence of trauma. Women who have sustained no serious injuries and are too early in their pregnancy to have a viable infant may be discharged directly from the emergency room. Observation with fetal monitoring on an obstetrical unit is recommended for any woman who is further along in her pregnancy.

In summary, we as health care workers need to get the word out that passenger restraint systems are essential for everyone. For our pregnant patients, one seat belt may have the effect of saving two lives. Enough said.

REFERENCES

Arneson S, Beltz E, Hahnemann B, Smith R. Automobile seat belt practices of pregnant women. *J Obstet Gynecol Neonatal Nurs* Jul–Aug; 15(4): 339–44, 1986.

Attico NB, Smith RJ, Fitzpatrick MB, Keneally M. Automobile safety restraints for pregnant women and children. *J Reprod Med* Mar; 31(3): 187–92, 1986.

Automobile passenger safety education for pregnant women and infants. Attitudes and practices of obstetrician-gynecologists. *J Reprod Med* Nov; 30(11): 849–53, 1985.

Hammond TL, Mickens-Powers BF, Strickland D, Hankins GD. The use of automobile safety restraint systems during pregnancy. *J Obstet Gynecol Neonatal Nurs* 1990 Jul–Aug; 19(4): 339–43.1990.

Hendly GW, Votey SR. Injuries in restrained motor vehicle accident victims. *Ann Emerg Med* Jul; 24(1): 77–84, 1994.

Lane PL. Traumatic fetal deaths. *J Emerg Med* Sep–Oct; 7(5): 433–35, 1989.

Wolf ME, Alexander BH, Rivara FP, Hickok DE. A retrospective cohort study of seat belt use and pregnancy outcome after a motor vehicle crash. *J Trauma* Jan; 34(1): 116-9, 1993.

QUESTION: Can taking vitamins during early pregnancy prevent birth defects?

A. Yes. It is a proven fact that vitamins prevent birth defects—especially neural tube defects such as spina bifida.

B. Studies suggest that folic acid, which is one component of a prenatal vitamin, may prevent neural tube defects, but this is not a proven fact.
C. Vitamins help pregnant women feel better but don't really have anything to do with birth defects.
D. Vitamins have been shown to play a crucial role in preventing genetic problems in babies.

ANSWER: B.

For many years it has been known that pregnant women need extra iron. The reason for this increased iron requirement is that little junior acts like a fetal sponge and soaks up as much of mom's iron as possible to make blood cells for himself (or herself). If extra iron isn't consumed by women during pregnancy, their blood counts can steadily drop. During delivery, the average woman loses half a liter of blood, and if she already has a "low tank of gas" due to lack of iron, transfusions may be needed to avoid disaster. That is why most women are supplemented with prenatal vitamins containing large amounts of iron during pregnancy.

There are two problems with prenatal vitamins, however, that make them somewhat difficult to take. First of all, the large volume of iron makes many women rather nauseated. This nausea may be especially bothersome in the first trimester when many women are already nauseated due to the large amount of hormones released by the placenta during these three months. To avoid some of the nausea associated with vitamins, most of my patients take them either at night before sleep or with a meal. *(For all of you pharmacists out there, I know full well that taking prenatal vitamins on an empty stomach is ideal for maximum absorption into the bloodstream. For pregnant women, however, it is far better to take them with a meal and keep them down than it is to have them come back at you because of an empty stomach).* Secondly, vitamins can lead to big-time constipation. Therefore many women need stool softeners or extra fiber to offset this problem.

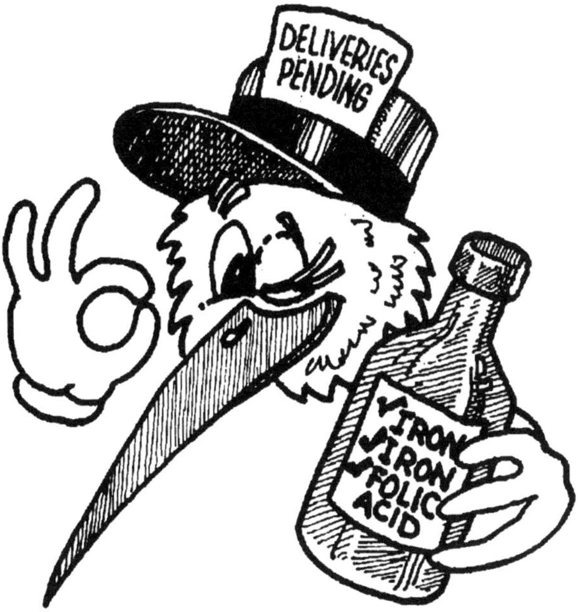

Besides keeping mom's blood count reasonable, is there any benefit to the baby in regard to preventing birth defects? A number of years ago it was noticed in animals that if drugs were given to decrease folic acid levels, their offspring were frequently born with brain or spinal cord abnormalities—so-called neural tube defects. That led researchers to see if they could decrease the incidence of neural tube defects in humans by giving folic acid. In 1989, Milunsky reviewed 23,491 pregnancies and divided women into two groups—those who took vitamins with folic acid, and those who did not. The incidence of neural tube defects was three times higher in the group that lacked folic acid. In 1994, the British Research Council published a study where 1,817 women who had previously delivered a child with a neural tube defect were followed throughout their entire pregnancy. The study took place over eight years and involved 33 centers. These women were given folic acid, vitamins, both, or neither during their pregnancy. It was found that folic acid, when taken before conception, greatly reduced the incidence of neural tube defects in this high risk group of women. This also led to the current recommendation that all women who are considering pregnancy take 0.4 mg of folic acid per day at least one month before conception and that women with previous children who have neural tube defects take 4 mg per day. Most prescription prenatal vitamins have 1 mg. In fact, that is what makes the prescription necessary—if they have less than 1 mg., they may be sold over the counter.

Even though the above evidence looks pretty convincing for using folic acid to reduce neural tube defects in infants, there have been other studies that have failed to show a benefit. Because prenatal vitamins are fairly innocuous drugs, however, most physicians today follow the recommendations that all pregnant women should be on prenatals—preferably before conception. There appears to be little risk with their use and some potentially significant benefits.

REFERENCES

British Medical Research Council Vitamin Study Research Group: Prevention of neural tube defects. Results of the medical research council vitamin study. *Lancet* 338: 131, 1991.

Cunningham FG, MacDonald, PC, Gant, NF, Leveno, KJ, Gilstrap LC. *Williams Obstetrics.* Appleton & Lange. Norwalk, Conn. 19th edition. 1993. pp. 259–60.

Milunsky A, Jick H, Jick SS, Bruell CL, MacLaughlin KS, Rothman KJ, Willett W: Multivitamin/folic acid supplementation in early pregnancy reduces the prevalence of neural tube defects. *JAMA* 262: 2847, 1989.

QUESTION: Are nausea and vomiting during pregnancy harmful to the baby?

A. Yes. Even mild nausea and vomiting can lead to significant malnutrition in the developing baby.

B. Yes. Even mild symptoms are dangerous, but only if they occur in the first trimester.

C. Essentially, no. Babies receive adequate nutrition from their mothers even when the mothers are nutritionally deprived during episodes of nausea and vomiting.

D. Babies born to women who experience a great deal of nausea and vomiting during their pregnancy are actually better off than other babies as this deprivation "toughens them up" for later in life.

ANSWER: C.

For about half of all you women out there, pregnancy is not only a time of great joy, but an opportunity to reacquaint yourself with the bathroom toilet bowl. It means spending countless hours fixing meals that you'll never eat and then spending the rest of the day kneeling before that great porcelain monument to misery. What causes all of this nausea during pregnancy, why do some women experience it while others don't, and how is junior faring through all of this commotion?

The nausea that some women experience during pregnancy is probably due to hormones produced by the placenta. For those of you who really care, they are human chorionic gonadotropin and estrogen. During early pregnancy, these hormone levels are rising rapidly and seem to be associated with the symptoms of nausea. Once the first trimester (or first three months of pregnancy) is up, the production of these hormones is not as great and most women notice that their nausea subsides. For a few unlucky souls, however, this nausea continues throughout the pregnancy. Fortunately, this continued queasiness is not common. And why do some women experience nausea and others don't?...well, it beats me. Let's just say that some women seem more sensitive to these hormones than others. That sounds as good as any explanation I can find in the literature.

In 1985, Klebanoff followed over 9000 women throughout their pregnancies, and made some observations concerning nausea and vomiting. First of all, he noticed that 56 percent of all of these women had nausea severe enough to actually vomit during their pregnancy. He then divided the women into two groups: those who experienced vomiting, and those who didn't. Interestingly, women who vomited tended to be younger, less educated, nonsmokers, and weighed more than women who did not have vomiting. When their pregnancy outcomes were analyzed, the group that experienced more vomiting had a lower miscarriage rate, a lower stillbirth rate, a lower premature birth rate, and there was no difference between the two groups with regard to infant birth weight. In other words, the overall outcome for the babies born to the mothers who tended to have nausea and vomiting during their pregnancy was actually better than the group that had no vomiting. Does this mean that women who have no vomiting are at higher risk than those who do? I certainly don't think so. What this study does imply, however, is that nausea and vomiting are not harmful to the baby.

You might be wondering how the fetus does so well in spite of all this nausea and vomiting. Basically, a baby can be compared to a little parasite. *(You actually don't really understand the true meaning of the parasite concept until they reach the teen years when they eat for an army and college tuition bills are due.)* He or she will get what they need despite the fact that mom is nutritionally deprived. This concept is strikingly obvious to physicians who have worked in third world countries where starvation is prevalent. Babies born to emaciated mothers who are in a state of starvation actually appear relatively plump and well nourished at the time of birth. Of course, the nutritional state of the baby usually deteriorates rather quickly after birth unless nutrition is available for the mother who is breast feeding, or for the baby if bottle feeding is used. The reason for this sparing of the newborn at the mother's expense is probably a survival mechanism that has worked for thousands of years to aid in propagating our species.

If nausea and vomiting are not harmful to the pregnancy and are relatively common, what can women do to make these symptoms more tolerable? First of all, the key to doing well during the first trimester is to keep well hydrated. This means drinking lots of clear liquids like Sprite or Kool-Aid. Why clear liquids? These fluids are absorbed quickly in the gastrointestinal tract and don't linger around in the bowel to cause nausea. Liquids that aren't clear such as milk, coffee, or orange juice are terribly nauseating and should be avoided like the plague. Once a woman is well hydrated, the nausea usually subsides enough to allow solid food to be eaten. This solid food should consist of bland foods such as potatoes or dry cereal. *(The Taco Bell specials and grandma's eye-watering gut-check chili should be enjoyed at a later time in the pregnancy.)* If a woman can't keep clear liquids down for 24 hours or so, then anti-nausea medicine such as promethazine suppositories may be used. These slippery little fellas can usually relieve the nausea long enough to allow hydration with clear liquids and stem the tide of the nausea. If the suppositories don't do the trick, then hydration with intravenous fluids at a hospital or at home by a home health care team is needed. How can a woman tell if she is hydrating herself appropriately? She can follow her urine production. The more she is urinating and the more dilute it is, the better hydrated she is. If she is urinating less often and has more concentrated urine, she needs to hydrate more. *(I bet you never thought urine could be so important, did you?)*

Is there some way that nausea and vomiting can actually be beneficial to a pregnancy? Nobody really knows. It seems as though there must be something good that comes out of this pregnancy-related nausea since it's so common. There are many theories as to why nausea may be beneficial in pregnancy, and my favorite one goes something like this: The first trimester is a time when all of the major organ systems are forming. These developing organs are very sensitive to foreign chemicals at this stage of life. If a pregnant woman were to ingest a harmful substance at this early time, it is more likely to harm the developing baby than if it is consumed later in pregnancy. Therefore the pregnant woman's body puts her in a state where she is less likely to ingest these chemicals by placing her in a state of nausea. Pretty neat theory, huh? Is there any hard evidence to support it? Nope. It is interesting but hard to prove and will probably always remain an imaginative thought.

The bottom line is that even though mom's *blowin' chow* to beat the band, little junior is enjoying life to its fullest. All his (or her) meals are brought around the clock, the thermostat is carefully controlled so that clothes aren't necessary, the room is dimly lit for sleeping comfort, and swimming is an option 24 hours a day. What more could a kid ask for?

REFERENCES

Cunningham FG, MacDonald PC, Gant NF, Leveno KJ, Gilstrap LC. *Williams Obstetrics*. 19th ed. Appleton & Lange. pp. 1146–7, 1993.

Klebanoff MA, Koslowe PA, Kaslow R, Rhoads GG. Epidemiology of vomiting in early pregnancy. *Obstet Gynecol* Nov; 66(5): 612–6, 1985.

QUESTION: Can the frequent use of ultrasounds during pregnancy be harmful to the baby?

A. Yes. The effects of ultrasounds on the developing baby are cumulative over time so that the more you do, the greater the chance of injury.
B. Yes. Ultrasounds affect the part of the brain that deals with good judgment, and your baby may be doomed to be an obstetrician when he or she grows up.
C. Only if the baby is listening when you are using the ultrasound.
D. No. To date, there are no studies that show any negative effects of ultrasounds in humans when they are used during pregnancy.

ANSWER: D.

I certainly hope that the answer is no. Otherwise my kids are in big trouble. There is no doubt that the ultrasound machine is one of the most utilized (and sometimes overutilized) pieces of equipment in obstetrics today. It is used early in pregnancy to verify both viability and dates, and later in pregnancy for many reasons including making the diagnosis of twins (or triplets or more), ensuring good growth, and picking up fetal abnormalities. It's a rare pregnancy today that is not evaluated at least once by this procedure.

What exactly is an ultrasound and is it really safe to use during pregnancy? An ultrasound is a machine that emits sound waves from a hand-held device. These sound waves are bounced off of all the tissues within the uterus and then a picture is formed on a TV-like screen. What appears on the screen is a picture of a "slice" through the uterus. By looking at many of these slices, a general picture of the pregnancy can be obtained. The safety of these ultrasound waves is related to the intensity of the wave. More intense waves tend to vibrate the tissues to a greater degree, which leads to heat production. This heat can be damaging to the surrounding tissues. In one study, for example, high intensity ultrasound waves were found to be damaging to the delicate tissues in the ears of mice. *(I wonder how you actually go about evaluating mice for loss of hearing? Maybe you sneak up behind them, yell CAT!!!, and observe their reaction).* Studies such as this one used ultrasound intensities much higher than those of traditional ultrasound. As a general rule, ultrasound levels less than 100 mW per cm^2 are considered safe and ultrasound equipment today currently use levels of 10 to 20 mW per cm^2.

Even though the immediate effects of ultrasounds on the fetus seem to be harmless, what about long-term effects? Lyons and co-workers followed 149 children who were exposed to ultrasounds during pregnancy and compared them to their siblings who were not exposed. The study followed these children for six years and found no negative developmental effects in these children compared to their brothers and sisters.

To summarize, then, there have been no long-term or short-term problems seen to date in children exposed to ultrasound sound waves. (This also holds true for the hand-held device called a Doppler that your physician or midwife uses to listen to the baby's heart beat during most visits. A Doppler also uses sound waves, but rather than forming a picture, the waves are amplified and heard through a speaker). *By the way, if you see any mice running around with hearing aids let them know that the researchers feel awful about the outcome of their study.*

REFERENCES

Creasy RK, Resnik R. *Maternal Fetal Medicine.* Third edition. WB Saunders Co. Phila., Pa. p. 203, 1994.

Cunningham FG, MacDonald PC, Gant NF, Leveno KJ, Gilstrap LC. *Williams Obstetrics.* 19th edition. Appleton & Lange. Norwalk, Conn. p. 987, 1993.

Lyons EA, Dyke C, Cheang M. In utero exposure to diagnostic ultrasound: A Six year follow-up. *Radiology* Mar; 166(3): 687–90, 1988.

Reece EA, Assimakopoulos E, Zheng XZ, Hagay Z, Hobbins JC. The safety of obstetric ultrasound: Concern for the fetus. *Obstet Gynecol* 76: 139, 1990.

QUESTION: Are caffeine and Nutrasweet harmful to use during pregnancy?

A. Caffeine can safely be used in moderate amounts, but Nutrasweet should be avoided.
B. Caffeine should be avoided, but Nutrasweet can be used safely in moderate amounts.
C. Caffeine can safely be used in moderate amounts, and Nutrasweet has never been shown to be harmful in pregnancy.
D. Both caffeine and Nutrasweet have been shown to be harmful in pregnancy and should be avoided in any dose.

ANSWER: C.

When subjects such as smoking and pregnancy or alcohol and pregnancy are brought up, there is usually little controversy. There might be a few of you who have lived in a hut in Bora Bora for the last 20 years and have not heard of the evils of smoking and alcohol, but most reasonable people have grasped the general concept that you should avoid these no no's during pregnancy. But as the subject turns to that staple food that we all know and love—*DIET COKE*—there seems to be a little more confusion. By the time many of my patients have made it in for their first prenatal visit, most women have decaffeinated and deNutrasweetened *(is that really a word?)* themselves. Quite to my surprise, many more women than you might expect continue to smoke, but very few of them continue their morning coffee or cola rituals. Quite a few of these women are a bit sheepish when they admit that they are still wrestling with their nicotine habit, but almost all are quite proud in telling you that they have been totally devoid of caffeine and artificial sweeteners from the second they found out they were pregnant. What exactly is the evidence for the dangers of caffeine and Nutrasweet during pregnancy?

As I stated above, the evils of smoking and persistent alcohol use during pregnancy are well known. The literature is loaded with overwhelming evidence of growth restriction, premature births, and fetal losses due to smoking, and permanent physical and intellectual impairments from chronic alcohol abuse during pregnancy. (By the way, another frequently asked question is, "Is it harmful to have an occasional glass of wine or an occasional cigarette?" The answer to this is, "Probably not," but it is very hard to draw the line between what is harmful and what is safe. Is a glass of wine per week okay? What about a glass per day? Because no one really knows where this cutoff is, I tend to make the blanket statement to just avoid alcohol during pregnancy.) When it comes to caffeine and Nutrasweet (or aspartame as it is medically known), there seems to be more myth than fact out there.

First let's tackle Nutrasweet because its easier. To date, there are no reports of adverse effects of Nutrasweet on the fetuses of pregnant women in humans or in laboratory animals. Even when you take families of mice who are expecting and give them a year's supply of their favorite diet soft drink, a TV (a small Japanese model fits the bill nicely), and all of the cheese doodles they can eat, their kids come out just fine. In some of these studies, the mice could drink no liquids without Nutrasweet, and still their kids were eventually accepted into the hallways of ivy league schools. *(We had a scare for a year or two when a higher proportion than usual went downhill intellectually and went into obstetrics and gynecology, but we found this to be only a momentary trend that corrected itself in later years.)*

For caffeine, the picture is a little muddier, but I think we are nearing a general consensus. The literature contains numerous studies that look at the relationship between caffeine and pregnancy. Some of the older studies suggest that caffeine may be linked to growth restriction, premature births, increased miscarriage rates, and infertility. The problem with most of these studies is they failed to account for other factors such as smoking and alcohol use. More recent studies that correct for these factors show low or moderate use (such as a cup or two of coffee per day) is probably not linked to these adverse outcomes. Heavy caffeine consumption, on the other hand, is linked to infant caffeine withdrawal (irritability, excessive crying, and sleeplessness), low birth weights, and poor fetal outcomes in general. (Maybe some of you have experienced caffeine withdrawal when you do something like visit Aunt Susie who has single-handedly decided to decaffeinate your entire family. On the first day you get a nagging headache. This is followed by some tremors, irritability, and constipation. By about the fourth or fifth day your entire family is at each other's throats, and you would gladly trade any of them in for even a lukewarm cup of three-day-old regular coffee. This is what newborns of heavy coffee drinkers go through.) Therefore I advise pregnant women to keep their caffeine consumption to a reasonable level throughout their pregnancy. Total elimination of all caffeine products including tea, cola, and chocolate, however, is unwarranted.

REFERENCES

Florack EI, Zielhuis GA, Rolland R. Cigarette smoking, alcohol consumption, and caffeine intake and fecundability. *Prev Med* Mar; 23(2): 175–80, 1994.

Godel JC, Pabst HF, Hodges PE, Johnson KE, Froese GJ, Joffres MR. Smoking and caffeine and alcohol intake during pregnant in a northern population: effect on fetal growth. *Can Med Assoc J* 147:181–8, 1992.

Mills JL, Holmes LB, Aarons JH, Simpson JL, Brown ZA, Jovanovic-Peterson LG, Conley MR, Graubard BI, Knopp RH, Metzger BE. Moderate caffeine use and the risk of spontaneous abortion and intrauterine growth retardation. *JAMA* Feb 3; 269(5): 593–7, 1993.

Pastore LM, Savitz DA. Case control study of caffeinated beverages and preterm delivery. *Am J Epidemiol* Jan 1; 141(1): 61–9, 1995.

Shu XO, Hatch MC, Mills J, Clemens M, Susser M. Maternal smoking, alcohol drinking, caffeine consumption, and fetal growth: results from a prospective study. *Epidiology* Mar; 6(2): 115–20, 1995.

Sivak A. Coteratogenic effects of caffeine. *Regul Toxicol Pharmacol* Feb; 19(1): 1–13, 1994.

William J H, Gayleen ME. Common questions patients ask during pregnancy. *Am Fam Physician* May 1: 51(6) 1465–70, 1995.

Yost DA. Clinical safety of aspartame. *Am Fam Physician* 39(2): 201–6, 1989.

Myths & Facts of Fetal Loss

As I mentioned in the Introduction, this chapter was placed here in the hope that it might provide some comfort to couples who have experienced a pregnancy loss—especially those who have gone through a miscarriage. I'm sure you can tell by now that I am usually a fairly upbeat kind of guy, but every once in a while you have to get serious. Now is one of those times. So excuse me if I get a bit preachy, but some of these concepts will hopefully be of value to some of you.

QUESTION: Do activities such as lifting heavy objects or riding roller coasters lead to miscarriage early in pregnancy?

A. No. Activities such as lifting or riding amusement rides have nothing to due with miscarrying.
B. Definitely.
C. Only if the activities involve lifting more than ten pounds.
D. Physical activities have nothing to due with miscarrying, but mentally stressful things do.

ANSWER: A.

This answer is an unequivocal NO!!! Women cannot control whether or not they will miscarry. At the time of conception, certain genetic and hormonal events occur that determine whether or not a pregnancy will be lost or continued, and activity has nothing to do with this.

First of all the definition of miscarriage is the loss of a pregnancy within the first half of a pregnancy—before the fetus is viable. Of all women who come to the office early in their pregnancy, approximately 15 percent will miscarry. The actual miscarriage rate is probably twice that (or around 30 percent) if you consider all of the women who miscarry so early that they don't even know they are pregnant. These women may bleed a little heavier or a little later than usual and may just assume that they had a "strange period." Around 80 percent of all of the miscarriages that occur are in the first three months of pregnancy.

Most miscarriages are caused by a genetic misalignment when the egg and sperm come together on the day of conception. This misalignment leads to a genetically abnormal fetus which doesn't develop normally. In many miscarriages the development of the fetus stops so early that there is no visible sign of the fetus—just an empty sac. Unfortunately, the placental tissue continues to develop for a while and it is this tissue that puts out the hormone that causes the nausea, headaches, and breast tenderness. This hormone (known as human chorionic gonadotropin or HCG for short) is also what is measured in our pregnancy tests and gives us a positive test. So for a while, we are all fooled into thinking the pregnancy is normal as a woman "feels pregnant" and our tests confirm the pregnancy. Somewhere down the line, however, (usually within the first three months) the body senses that there is no fetus and then the bleeding and cramping start. The cramping is due to uterine contractions as the uterus tries to empty itself of this placental tissue. Once the placental tissue has been expelled, the body is free to ovulate again and go about the business of getting pregnant. Please remember that this genetic misalignment is the reason most women miscarry. A small percentage of women will miscarry due to reasons such as a misshapen uterus or inadequate hormone production from the ovaries. They tend to have repeated miscarriages and need a medical evaluation to achieve successful future pregnancies. Fortunately, these types of miscarriages are very rare and are usually detected after a woman repeatedly miscarries.

To summarize, *PEOPLE DO NOT CAUSE MISCARRIAGES!* The outcome is "in the cards" from the day of conception, but we are not smart enough to figure it out until we start investigating with things like ultrasounds and hormone levels. So despite what grandma and Aunt Susie say, it is not what you do that makes you miscarry. Back in grandma's time, she might have remembered that right before she miscarried, she picked up something heavy and she assumed that her lifting "caused" the miscarriage. The miscarriage was destined to happen. Unfortunately, everyone remembers something they did before they miscarried. As I tell my patients, once conception occurs, they are just "along for the ride." That's why most physicians don't place women on activity restrictions early in pregnancy anymore.

As a physician, it is easy for me to understand that miscarriage is nature's way of assuring that the overwhelming majority of kids that we humans have will be normal. In other words, most of the genetic miscues are eliminated very early in the reproductive process. To the woman who is miscarrying, however, this whole process is viewed very differently. She usually understands mentally that the miscarriage is all for the best, but emotionally it is quite a different story. You see, as soon as most women realize they are pregnant, they envision their baby growing up straight and strong, going to school, and leading a life of which she can be proud. When the reality of the miscarriage hits, it can be emotionally devastating. This woman needs the support of family, friends, and her medical caregiver, but this help needs to be channeled in the right direction. She understands some of the ideas I have previously outlined, but most of all she needs to understand that she did absolutely nothing to cause the loss of her pregnancy. This will help out when well-meaning but misguided friends and relatives imply it was something she did that caused this event. And for heaven's sake, don't tell this woman she can start over again. She doesn't want to start over again...at least not now. She has just had a major loss in her life and needs to work through the grieving process. Try to avoid any comments in regard to the cause of her loss and just be there for her. Let her know that you will help her work through this tough time in her life and that you will also be there later to share in the good times.

REFERENCES

Creasy RK, Resnick R. *Maternal Fetal Medicine.* Third edition. WB Saunders Co. Philadelphia, Pa. pp. 35–6.

Cunningham FG, MacDonald PC, Gant NF, Leveno KJ, Gilstrap LC. *Williams Obstetrics.* 19th edition. Appleton and Lange. Norwalk, Conn. pp. 665–78.

QUESTION: Does vaginal bleeding during early pregnancy mean that you will miscarry?

A. Yes. Vaginal bleeding always indicates that a miscarriage will occur.
B. Usually. Once vaginal bleeding has occurred, only rarely does a woman avoid a miscarriage.
C. Either a miscarriage or a normal pregnancy is possible, and further testing can distinguish between the two.
D. No. Vaginal bleeding is a normal part of pregnancy and miscarriage rarely occurs.

ANSWER: C.

It is important to understand that vaginal bleeding is not always bad. In fact, when vaginal bleeding occurs early in pregnancy, miscarriage results only about half of the time. Some examples of bleeding in a normal pregnancy are as follows: 1) During pregnancy, the blood supply to the uterus is greatly increased. The cervix, or the opening of the uterus, lies in the back of the vagina. Sometimes small vessels in the cervix can break down and bleed either during intercourse or for no good reason at all. This bleeding usually stops after a few hours or days and the pregnancy proceeds normally. 2) The placenta is a large vascular organ that is attached to the inside of the uterus and supplies the baby with good home-cooked meals and plenty of oxygen. Early in pregnancy this organ may be found overlying the cervix. Since the placenta is very vascular, it may bleed a little, and this blood may exit through the cervix and vagina. As the pregnancy progresses, the placenta usually moves away from the cervix and this bleeding stops. The pregnancy then proceeds normally. Rarely, the placenta might cover the cervix throughout the entire pregnancy and a Caesarean section would be needed to prevent large amounts of blood loss during delivery. These two examples are mentioned to illustrate how vaginal bleeding may lead to a normal outcome.

What every pregnant woman fears, of course, when she bleeds is that she is miscarrying. As you learned in the last segment, miscarriages usually occur when there is a genetic misalignment at the time of conception. More rarely, there may be things like uterine abnormalities and hormonal deficiencies that may also lead to miscarriage. When a woman has vaginal bleeding early in pregnancy, how then can you tell if she will miscarry or proceed with a normal pregnancy?

First of all, a pelvic ultrasound may give you some valuable information. Beginning about six weeks from the first day of a woman's last menstrual period, a fetus with a heartbeat can be seen on ultrasound. When a fetus is seen, it is fairly reassuring that things are all right. Sometimes there can be some early development before a miscarriage, but for the most part, visualization of a fetus on ultrasound is a pretty good sign that the bleeding is not due to miscarriage. Most genetic misalignments cause the fetus to be lost so early that there is no more evidence of it and only an empty sac is seen. Once you see this sac, you know either that this is a miscarriage (commonly called a blighted ovum) or that the pregnancy is just too early to see the fetus. Is there a way to distinguish between a blighted ovum and an early normal pregnancy? Certainly—by using hormone levels.

A hormone called human chorionic gonadotropin or HCG is secreted by the placenta during pregnancy. This is the same hormone that we detect in pregnancy tests to tell if a woman is pregnant. In a normal pregnancy, this hormone level doubles every other day. So if blood is drawn and a level of 1000 is obtained on a Monday, then on Wednesday it should be 2000, on Friday it should be 4000 and so on. If a woman is miscarrying, the levels tend to drop as the placental tissue stops producing the hormone. By using ultrasounds and hormone levels we can play a bit of a detective game and figure out whether women who are bleeding are going to miscarry or proceed with a normal pregnancy. Keep in mind that neither ultrasounds nor HCG levels (or anything else for that matter) can prevent pregnancy losses, but they can give a woman an idea of what to expect early in a pregnancy when she has vaginal bleeding.

By the way, another cause of vaginal bleeding early in pregnancy that I have not discussed is an ectopic pregnancy. This type of pregnancy occurs when the pregnancy develops outside of the uterus. The most common type of ectopic pregnancy is a tubal pregnancy. This occurs when an egg is released from the ovary and is fertilized in the tube by a sperm cell. The fertilized egg fails to make it out of the tube and implants in the tube and begins to grow. As it grows, the tube may rupture causing internal and/or vaginal bleeding. Tubal pregnancies are suspected when a pregnant woman has pelvic pain and bleeding early in pregnancy. On ultrasound there is no fetus in the uterus and sometimes a mass may be seen in the tube. When HCG levels are obtained, these levels tend to rise, but not as much as the doubling every other day that is seen with a normal pregnancy. Treatment of a tubal pregnancy involves surgically removing the pregnancy from the tube or removing the tube itself. *(No, we are not able to save the pregnancy and place it back in the uterus, but I'm glad to see that you are still awake. Maybe someday this type of transplant technology will be possible).*

REFERENCES

Creasy RK, Resnick R. *Maternal Fetal Medicine.* Third edition. WB Saunders Co. Philadelphia, Pa. pp. 35–6.

Cunningham FG, MacDonald PC, Gant NF, Leveno KJ, Gilstrap LC. *Williams Obstetrics.* 19th edition. Appleton and Lange. Norwalk, Conn. pp. 665–78.

QUESTION: Once it has been established that a woman is miscarrying, should she have a D & C done?

A. Yes. If she doesn't, the remaining tissue could lead to an infection.
B. No. Having a D & C will make her more likely to develop an infection.
C. No D & C's should really never be done. Nature will take care of things just fine.
D. Having a D & C or letting nature take its course are both acceptable ways of handling a miscarriage.

ANSWER: D.

Once it has been determined that a woman is miscarrying (either by physical examination, ultrasound, and/or hormone levels), a woman has basically two options: 1) having a D & C performed or 2) allowing her uterus to expel the remaining tissue on its own. Which option is appropriate depends on the woman and the situation. Let me explain this in a little more detail.

First of all, what exactly is a D & C? This is a surgical procedure that involves removing the placental tissue within the uterus (and any fetal tissue if it is present. Remember that many times there is only an empty sac when a miscarriage takes place.) This procedure involves giving a woman some type of anesthesia—either general anesthesia (commonly known as "going to sleep"), epidural anesthesia (which gets you numb from your waist on down), or intravenous medications (kind of like having one too many margaritas so that you know the procedure is being done, but you really don't care). Once the anesthesia is in place, the cervix (or bottom part of the uterus) is *dilated* with a series of probes that get progressively larger. (That's the "D" part). Then the tissue within the uterus is removed or *curetted* from the uterus. (That's the "C" part). The advantage of a D & C is that it puts an immediate end to the cramping and/or bleeding that a woman experiences when she is miscarrying. Sometimes this cramping and bleeding can go on for days or weeks, which can be pretty annoying or downright painful. The disadvantage of a D & C is that it is a surgical procedure and has some risks associated with it. These complications include infection, perforation, scarring, and the usual anesthetic risks associated with any surgical procedure. These risks rarely occur, but it is important to understand that any procedure has its potential problems.

The other option a woman has is to allow the uterine tissue to pass on its own. The obvious advantage is that she avoids any kind of surgical procedure and possible complications. The disadvantage is that passing this tissue involves cramping and bleeding that could persist for days or even weeks. If a woman elects this option, I see her in the office on a weekly basis to talk about how she is doing and to draw hormone (HCG or human chorionic gonadotropin) levels. These levels drop as a woman passes and/or reabsorbs the placental tissue (not all of the tissue has to be passed—some is simply reabsorbed by the body). Once these levels have dropped to zero, the cramping and bleeding can be expected to stop and ovulation will occur resulting in the resumption of periods.

In my practice, I explain these two options to couples who are experiencing a miscarriage and assure them that either is acceptable. As a general rule, the earlier a miscarriage takes place, the smaller the amount of tissue that is present and the easier it is to pass the tissue on your own. Miscarriages which take place late in the first trimester are more often associated with severe cramping and bleeding that require a D & C. I also explain that when a woman elects to pass the tissue on her own, she can always change her mind and have a D & C if the cramping and bleeding are more than what she can reasonably handle. It is also important to understand that an accurate diagnosis of a miscarriage must be made before these options are given. This avoids no-no's like waiting to pass tissue when in fact a woman has a tubal pregnancy, which needs to be surgically removed before the tube ruptures.

QUESTION: Can you can strangle your baby with its umbilical cord by placing your arms over your head?

A. Yes. Especially late in pregnancy when the umbilical cord is more fully developed.
B. Yes. This can occur any time in pregnancy.
C. Only with repeated arm movements over the head such as jumping jacks.
D. Absolutely not. This is an absurd and potentially harmful myth.

ANSWER: D.

I am writing this while sitting in our basement family room on a cold winter day in February. Later on today I will be attending a funeral for a baby I delivered earlier in the week for one of my patients. She was approaching her due date and called me late one evening after not feeling the baby move for a few hours. Upon arrival at the hospital, no fetal heart tones could be heard, and an ultrasound verified that the baby had died. This scenario is one that most obstetricians have experienced and all dread. Of course the patient is always the model patient who takes great care of herself and has never missed a visit—even when it meant fighting through two-foot snow drifts to make her last appointment.

At the time of delivery, a tight cord was found around the baby's neck. In my discussions with the family, I emphasized that "cord accidents" such as this one are impossible to prevent despite all of our modern technology. "You will think of about a thousand things that you did over the past few days," I said, "but none of them had anything to do with these recent events." Despite all of the anguish that goes along with losing a child, I could see some momentary comfort for my patient in these words. You see, I knew that at least one of her well-intentioned relatives had already quizzed her on her recent activities such as reaching over her head. It's only human nature to think that any event, whether it is good or bad, is directly under our control. Unfortunately, many are not.

So how common is it that a baby is delivered with a cord around its neck and does it relate to a mother moving her extremities? The answers are VERY and NO! In a study by Dr. Gary Hankins involving 1,000 consecutive deliveries, more than 20 percent had cords around the neck and there were no fetal deaths. This really is considered a normal finding at delivery. Fortunately it is extremely rare to have the cord become so tight that it impedes blood flow through it and causes fetal death. When this does occur it is immensely important to reassure women that these types of events are totally beyond their control. Most of all, we need to avoid propagating this hurtful myth. To reiterate, movements of your extremities have nothing to due with a baby's umbilical cord.

REFERENCES

Hankins GVD, Snyder RR, Hauth JC, Gilstrap LC III, Hammond T: Nuchal cords and neonatal outcome. *Obstet Gynecol* 70: 687 1987.

QUESTION: Is having a "tipped" or "tilted" uterus associated with problems such as infertility, miscarriage, and pelvic pain?

A. Yes. This condition needs immediate surgical correction.
B. Yes, but it only leads to problems in about half of all women.
C. Yes, mainly infertility. In fact, women who have this type of uterus need to have intercourse while standing on their heads if they want to conceive.
D. No. The position of the uterus has nothing to do with infertility, miscarriage, pelvic pain, or any other problems for that matter.

ANSWER: D.

I had just finished Mary's pap smear and was starting to do the second part of the pelvic exam. This involves feeling vaginally with one hand and abdominally with the other to asses the uterus and ovaries. "Oh yes," Mary interjected, "Someone told me that I have a tipped uterus. Is that bad? I've heard that it's harder to get pregnant and easier to lose a pregnancy with a tipped uterus." The answer to this question is a hardy "NOT!"

Between 10 and 20 percent of all women have a retroverted or retroflexed uterus. What this means is that when we feel for the uterus on pelvic exam, these women have a uterus that arches backward toward the rectum as opposed to the other 80 to 90 percent of women whose uteri curve upward toward the abdomen. It's a little like being left-handed. Most people are right-handed, but being left-handed carries no negative connotation except that left handers have inferior intellect *(just kidding...calm down all you lefties).*

Does having a retroverted uterus make you more prone to infertility, pregnancy loss, or pelvic pain? No, no, and no again. In my literature search back to 1966, I could only find one study that implied anything negative in regard to a retroverted uterus. Weeks et. al. found a 16 percent miscarriage rate compared to 9 percent for other women. This difference is small and I could find no other studies to back this up. There is one condition, however, that rarely occurs with women who have a retroverted uterus. This is where the uterus gets entrapped against the sacrum (or "tail bone") early in pregnancy as it grows. This tends to lift and rotate the cervix upward and block the urethra. Typically, women who develop this condition wake up in the morning and during their usual trip to the bathroom, find that they can't urinate. The patient usually calls rather frantically; her bladder is approximately the size of a beach ball, but urination is impossible. In the office, a catheter may be inserted into the urethra, past the obstruction, and into the bladder. This drains the bladder giving the patient immediate relief and makes you the doctor a popular person. The next thing that needs to be done is to place the woman in a knee–chest position (in other words with her rear end up in the air) and then vaginally try to dislodge the entrapped uterus. (Sounds pretty weird, huh?) Sometimes this works in the office, and other times anesthesia is needed to relax the poor patient so the uterus can be forced up out of the pelvis. Once the uterus has been lifted out of the pelvis and into the lower abdomen, it usually cannot become entrapped again. So far in four years of residency and thirteen years of practice, I have had this happen to two of my obstetrical patients. Both times anesthesia was needed to relieve this condition. Most likely this was due to my wimpiness to press hard enough to force the uterus into the proper position in an unanesthetized (try saying that fast three times) patient in the office. By the way, trying to explain these weird maneuvers to a significant other in your office is a real trip. Generally, though, they are relieved to find that intercourse or related antics of the night before had nothing to do with their partner's condition.

Before I leave this subject, I would like to throw out another little tidbit of information. Remember when I said that I only had two "obstetrical" patients that were affected negatively by a retroverted uterus? Well, I actually had a non-pregnant patient who was referred to me by a family practitioner for evaluation of a urinary problem. Basically, she had to strain for hours each morning in order to urinate. On exam, she was found to have muscular tumors in her retroverted uterus that increased the size of the uterus to that of a four month pregnancy. Although these tumors were benign, they caused complete urinary retention, and the uterus could not be reduced even under anesthesia. Eventually she needed a hysterectomy (removal of the uterus) to cure the problem.

REFERENCES

Cunningham FG, MacDonald PC, Gant NF, Leveno KJ, Gilstrap LC. *Williams Obstetrics.* 19th edition. Appleton & Lange. Norwalk, Conn. pp. 531–2, 1993.

Weekes ARL, Atlay RD, Brown VA, Jordan EC, Murray SM. The retroverted gravid uterus and its effect on the outcome of pregnancy. *Br Med J* 1: 622, 1976.

Postpartum Myths & Facts

These myths and facts deal with issues that affect women after delivery. The major category here is breast feeding. Grandma and Aunt Susie are just full of advice to give you when you bring that bundle of joy home. Some of it might even be worthwhile. This chapter will examine a few of these issues.

QUESTION: For women who choose not to breast feed or for women who are weaning their infants, is there any medication that can keep them from getting breast engorgement?

A. Yes. There is a medication that works well for preventing breast engorgement immediately after delivery, and later for weaning.
B. Yes, but the medication works only when used immediately after delivery. It is not effective later on for weaning.
C. No. There is no approved medication, but breast binders and ice packs work nicely.
D. No. There is no approved medication, but large amounts of alcoholic beverages and biting on a bullet work pretty well.

ANSWER: C.

During my residency in the early 1980s, there were numerous medications on the market for the prevention of breast tenderness. Over time, all of these medications were seen to have more potential risks than benefits. Most of these medications fell into two groups: estrogens and bromocriptine. Estrogens had some suppressive effects on milk production when used immediately after delivery, but made pregnant women more prone to blood-clotting problems. Bromocriptine also suppressed lactation after delivery, but was fairly nauseating and was seen to cause extremely high blood pressure in a small number of women. Neither of these medications was effective in the suppression of breast engorgement after breast feeding was started—only when used immediately after delivery. Both groups of medications were taken off the market for the use of milk suppression after delivery due to their potentially serious side effects.

When these medications were first withdrawn from the market, a collective groan went up from the obstetricians in this country because we knew that we would be inundated with calls from miserable postpartum patients with breasts about to erupt. The only thing that we had to offer them was breast binders and ice packs. Much to my surprise, these calls did not occur. In fact, I can honestly say that the incidence of breast engorgement in my practice has not increased since the withdrawal of these drugs. Immediately after delivery, I have all of my non–breast feeding patients wear tight fitting bras 24 hours a day. The only time they remove them is to take a shower, but otherwise they are worn nonstop—even to sleep at night. If some engorgement does occur, they apply ice packs, which seem to control the swelling nicely. For breast feeding women who want to wean their infants, they decrease their feedings gradually while using ice packs and a tight-fitting bra. This seems to work pretty well provided they keep the weaning gradual.

The alcohol/bullet technique can be used if the above method fails, but has the distinct disadvantage of awful hangovers and potential dental injuries.

QUESTION: Are cabbage leaves good for treating breast tenderness?

A. You bet. This old-time remedy really works.
B. No, but they make a great fashion statement.
C. Cabbage leaves work only if they are chilled as it is the coolness of the leaves that relieves breast tenderness—the cabbage is probably unimportant.
D. The only thing chilled here are the brains of those who believe in this ridiculous wive's tale.

ANSWER: A.

For all of you investors out there, I've got a hot stock tip...cabbage leaf bras. Yeah, you heard me right, cabbage leaf bras. It's the latest, or should I say earliest fad for treating postpartum breast tenderness. Usually about two or three days after delivery, the breasts begin to produce milk as if there were no tomorrow. If junior isn't chowing down appropriately to keep up with this production or if a woman elects not to breast feed, mom may feel as if she has two volcanoes about to explode. Over the last few decades, numerous medications have been tried to reduce this monumental pain. As we discussed in the previous question, hormones like estrogen and hormone suppressants like bromocriptine have been used, but were stopped either due to lack of effectiveness or intolerable side effects or both. That leaves non–breast feeding women with breast binders and ice packs and breast feeding women with virtually nothing.

Don't tell grandma, but one of her old time remedies is coming back into vogue...cabbage leaves. Is there really any basis for the notion that these simple plants could lead to much needed mammiferous relief for new moms? *(Don't look that word up...I guarantee it isn't in your Funk and Wagnall's)*. In 1993, Nikodem et. al. took 120 breast feeding women 72 hours after delivery and placed them into two groups. One group was treated with cabbage leaves to their breasts and the other group received routine care. The cabbage leaf group had greater success with breast feeding as 76 percent of them were still breast feeding at six weeks compared to 58 percent of the control group. The experimenters admitted, however, that they weren't sure if the greater success of the cabbage leaf group was due to its medicinal value or due to a placebo effect.

Many believers in the cabbage leaf prophesy insist that the cabbage leaves need to be chilled. Could it be that it is merely the cold temperature that reduces the swelling and pain. To answer this question, Roberts et. al. in 1995 did a comparison of chilled versus room temperature cabbage leaves to reduce breast engorgement in breast feeding women. They took 28 lactating women with breast engorgement and randomized them to chilled or room temperature cabbage leaves, which were applied to the breasts for a two-hour period. Both groups reported significantly less pain at the end of the two hours, with absolutely no difference between these two groups. They concluded that chilling the cabbage leaves was not necessary. There seems to be some chemical or combination of chemicals within the leaf that soothes the breast and inhibits engorgement. There is also evidence that some of these same chemicals may actually prevent cancer (including breast cancer) in humans as well as animals. Just one more reason to eat your veggies, like mama told you so many years ago.

REFERENCES

Lust KD, Brown JE, Thomas W. Maternal intake of cruciferous vegetables and other foods and colic symptoms in exclusively breast fed infants. *J Am Diet Assoc* Jan; 96(1): 46–8, 1996.

Nikodem VC. Danziger D, Gebka N, Gulmezoglu AM, Hofmeyr GJ. Do cabbage leaves prevent breast engorgement? A randomized, controlled study. *Birth* June; 20(2): 61–4, 1993.

Roberts L, Reiter M, Schuster D. A comparison of chilled and room temperature cabbage leaves in treating breast engorgement. *J Hum Lact* Sep; 11(3): 1991–4, 1995.

Stoewsand GS. Bioactive organosulfur phytochemicals in Brassica oleracea vegetables—a review. *Food Chem Toxicol* June; 33(6): 537–43, 1995.

QUESTION: Is the birth of a baby an event that tends to bring a couple closer together?

A. You bet. Smelly diapers, baby puke, and late night feedings can be a real turn-on for couples with marital problems.
B. If bonding occurs between a man, a woman, and their baby immediately after birth, they should have no problems after delivery. Those couples who don't bond will usually have marital discord for a while.
C. Usually. Most relationships become closer, but the really troubled couples will drift apart after the birth of a child.
D. Usually not. The birth of a child is an event that brings many new pressures to a relationship and should never be used to mend a troubled one.

ANSWER: D.

Ah, yes...I remember it as though it were yesterday. It was four months since the birth of our first child and life was wonderful...well maybe not perfect...actually it was kind of the pits. I was lying on the couch in our family room after a particularly grueling couple of days of delivering babies at the hospital and reminiscing about the last several months. Our son was born unexpectedly three weeks early after my wife's water broke. *(What we were doing when it broke, I won't get into.)* Of course he was breech, which led to a Cesarean section after months of preparation with natural childbirth classes, but that was okay. He was just about the cutest thing we had ever seen. I remember laying him down in his crib after we arrived home from the hospital thinking, "Gee, what do we do now?" Well it didn't take us very long to figure it out. Between feeding, changing, and bathing the little guy, my wife didn't have time for much else. I, of course, was little help as I was either working at the hospital (as a resident at the time), or trying to get caught up on sleep. Between her schedule and mine, we hardly saw each other. Weeks went by and then months and I found myself lying on our living room couch thinking, "This is the wonderful life we were looking forward to for nine long months?"

This is a common scenario recounted to me by many of my patients. You see, our culture puts all of the emphasis on preparing for delivery, but very little on what happens afterward. Delivery is a drop in the bucket compared to what follows. We are all led to believe that if we can just make it through those nine months of bloating, nausea, and backache, the world will be our oyster. Well I've got news for you...It ain't so. The period of time after the birth of a child is probably the most difficult time of your life. It can be a strain on even the best of marriages.

From the guys' point of view, they have been very patient for nine months and now they want their wives back so they can enjoy some pampering of their own. Every time they approach their mate, however, she is always with the kid or is dead tired from being up all night. When she is not receptive to his advances because of sheer exhaustion, he feels unwanted and resentful of junior.

From the woman's point of view, she has no time of her own. She feels like a human milk machine that is continually sleep deprived and is totally at the mercy of this new addition. She wants to enjoy life like she used to, but is just too tired. Yes, indeed, kids are wonderful and most of us would gladly go through it all again *(as my wife and I did two other times),* but they are by no means a way to bring a couple together.

I see many couples who have grown apart after the birth of their child. Once they understand what is happening, they can work together to find time for themselves and reverse this downhill spiral. First of all, babies begin to sleep for longer periods of time which helps decrease the parent's sleep deprivation. Next, I advise couples to start with simple things like going for a walk in a mall together or having an occasional dinner out. Of course it helps if they have some dependable relatives to whom they can entrust their newborn. But for the well-being of the family, parents need to feel like a couple again and relearn to enjoy each other. Fortunately for most couples, this time of discord is short lived and they move on to better times. If it lingers, however, professional counseling may be necessary.

QUESTION: Does wine really help your milk come in when you are breast feeding?

A. Yes. Wine is extremely helpful in initiating breast feeding after delivery.
B. No. Wine actually interferes with your milk as it comes in and also can give it a taste that babies don't like.
C. Wine has no effect on moms or babies.
D. Who cares? It makes moms and babies so mellow that neither one usually complains.

ANSWER: B.

As we discussed in the last question, those first few days after delivery can be some of the most exasperating times of a woman's life. She has just expelled a humongous living being from her bottom (in the case of a vaginal delivery) or has had major abdominal surgery (in the case of a Cesarean section). She may have vaginal or abdominal stitches and undoubtedly has the worst case of hemorrhoids she can imagine. This whole process has probably made her sleep-deprived, and now she must care for an infant 24 hours a day as family and friends drop in on her at all hours. As she cradles her newborn infant in her arms, it is frightening to think that this little E.T.-like creature is totally dependent on her for survival. With this setting as a backdrop, it is no wonder many women "lose it" emotionally when they place their new bundle of joy to their breast and he or she falls asleep faster than I do at an opera. A great deal of folklore has evolved to aid women in these first few days after delivery. One of the more popular bits of advice women get involves drinking wine to enhance breast feeding. Let's investigate to see if there is some sound basis for this advice.

The general idea behind this notion is that wine triggers something called the letdown reflex. This reflex involves the contraction of tiny muscles around the nipple, which starts the milk flowing. This reflex can be initiated by the sucking of the infant or things that remind a woman of breast feeding such as the baby crying. When asked to describe what this feels like, many women describe it as a "pins-and-needles" sensation that is followed by the flowing of milk from the nipple. Wine, or so the myth goes, enhances this reflex and leads to increased milk production and a happier baby.

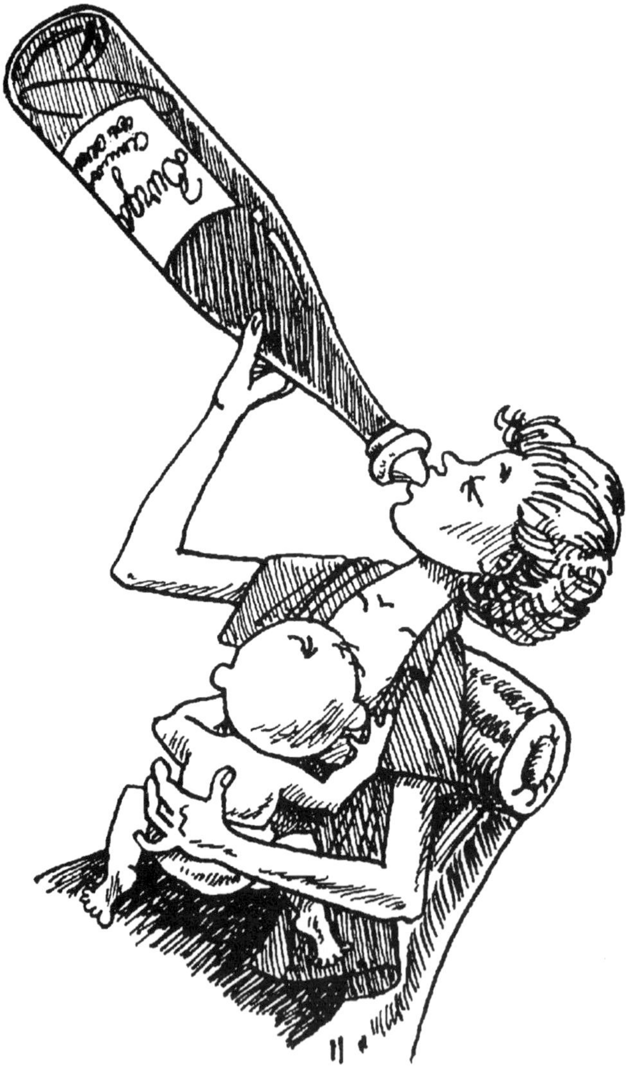

In animal studies, however, alcohol is seen to actually inhibit the letdown reflex. This makes sense if you think about it for a while. Alcohol has long been known to be a muscle relaxant. I remember spending long hours as a medical student on the high-risk obstetrical unit tending intravenous alcohol drips. The muscle relaxant effect of alcohol was used at that time to stop contractions in women who experienced premature labor. It probably didn't work all that well, but it sure made for happier patients. The detrimental effects of this drug on the fetus also made it a poor choice for anything but short-term treatment. When other safer and more effective drugs were discovered, alcohol was no longer prescribed for pregnant women. This same muscle relaxing quality of alcohol interferes with the small ejecting muscles of the breast and is a hindrance to breast feeding.

Alcohol not only interferes with milk ejection, but gets into the breast milk itself. In fact, the level of alcohol in the breast milk is equal to or greater than the level found in the breast feeding mother's blood. Of course this level of alcohol is further diluted out in the baby's bloodstream, but the bottom line is that alcohol certainly reaches the baby during breast feeding. Can these levels be detrimental to infants? In one study from the University of Michigan, 400 breast feeding infants were followed up to one year of age. Detailed histories were taken from the mothers of these infants including their alcohol intake while breast feeding. They used the Bayley Mental Development Index and the Psychomotor Development Index to evaluate each infant's mental and motor development. Their findings showed that exposing the infants to increasing amounts of alcohol had no effect on their mental development, but had a "slight but significant effect" on their motor development.

From the infant's point of view, does mom's consuming alcohol affect his or her desire to nurse? In one interesting study reported in the *New England Journal of Medicine* in 1991, twelve breast feeding women were studied to see how alcohol in their breast milk affected their infants. First of all, they drank orange juice containing alcohol and samples of their breast milk were collected at regular intervals. A panel of adults then smelled the breast milk samples to see if there was a change in odor. The samples were also analyzed for their alcohol content. The panel uniformly noticed that with increasing levels of alcohol, the intensity of a bad odor within the milk increased. Moreover, infants significantly decreased their nursing as the alcohol content of the milk increased. The increased intensity of the odor of the milk peaked between 30 minutes to one hour after consumption. Nursing during this time period decreased to the lowest levels of any time in the study.

It would appear, then, that the wine theory of breast feeding is a myth. After wine ingestion, the letdown reflex is decreased, the milk develops a strong odor, infants seem to feed less vigorously, and there may be some long-term negative effects on babies. Wasting away in Margaritaville may momentarily help mom forget about her aching bottom and assist in ending her sleep deprivation, but little junior will probably not be a happy camper if this treatment becomes routine.

REFERENCES

Davidson S, Alden L, Davidson P. Changes in alcohol consumption after childbirth. *J Adv Nurs* May; 6(3): 195–8, 1981.

Lawton ME. Alcohol in breast milk. *Aust N Z J Obstet Gynaecol* Feb; 25(1): 71–3, 1985.

Little RE, Anderson KW, Ervin CH, Worthington-Roberts B, Clarren SK. Maternal alcohol use during breast feeding and infant mental and motor development at one year. *N Engl J Med* Aug 17; 321(7): 425–30, 1989.

Mennella JA, Beauchamp GK. The transfer of alcohol to human milk. Effects on flavor and the infant's behavior. *N Engl J Med* Oct 3; 325(14); 981–5, 1991.

QUESTION: Can you get pregnant while you are breast feeding?

A. Nope. By the way...Could I interest you in some prime Florida swamp land?

B. It's possible, but as long as you haven't had a period, you are safe.

C. Ovulation among breast feeding women is highly variable—some women ovulate regularly, some irregularly, and some not at all. Pregnancy, though, is most definitely possible.

D. Not only is pregnancy possible, but women are actually more fertile while breast feeding than when they aren't.

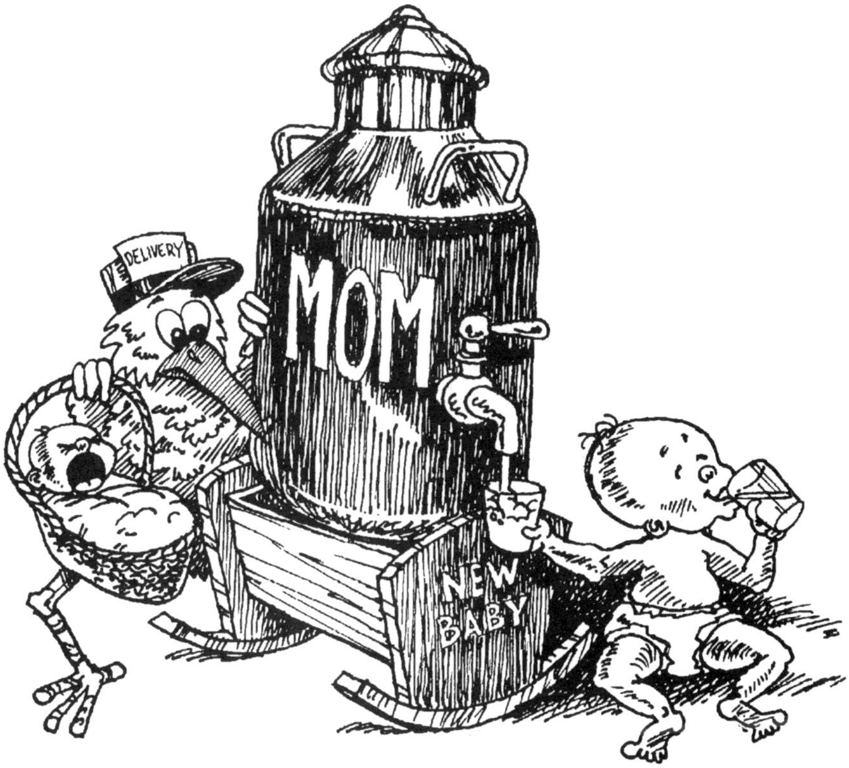

ANSWER: C.

Ah yes…a subject near and dear to the heart of many an obstetrician or midwife. At least those who like delivering lots of babies. As many of you know (some from first hand experience), this question may be answered by an unequivocal "Yes." In non–breast feeding women, ovulation may occur within four weeks of delivery. In breast feeding women, on the other hand, ovulation is usually delayed. The time interval between delivery and ovulation, however, is highly variable during lactation. Some women never have a period during the entire time they are breast feeding, while other women ovulate on a regular monthly basis. As a general rule, 50 to 75 percent of all breast feeding women will ovulate within 36 weeks of delivery. The bottom line is that ovulation is highly unpredictable in breast feeding women and pregnancy may result if this fact is forgotten.

I have also heard the comment "I will start using some kind of birth control when my first period begins." Remember that ovulation occurs first, and then bleeding results if no pregnancy occurs. My advice is to use some kind of birth control if a pregnancy is not desired. Also keep in mind that as the frequency of breast feeding decreases, normal cycles are more likely to resume.

REFERENCES

Precis V: An Update in Obstetrics and Gynecology. American College of Obstetrics and Gynecology. 1994. page 202.

QUESTION: Is it okay to take birth control pills when you are breast feeding?

A. Yes.
B. No.
C. Both yes and no.
D. You don't need birth control pills while breast feeding since you can't get pregnant.

ANSWER: C.

Yes and no?...How can that be?...No, I'm not pulling your leg *(or any other part of your anatomy for that matter)*. Let me explain. As I mentioned in a previous question, there are actually two types of birth control pills: 1) combination pills (or standard birth control pills), which contain estrogen and progesterone and 2) progesterone-only pills (also called the "mini-pill"). Both types of pills are very effective in preventing pregnancy and safe to use while breast feeding. The estrogen in the combination pills, however, suppresses the milk supply in nursing mothers. For this reason, most physicians shy away from combination pills during breast feeding. Progesterone-only pills are not only safe to use while breast feeding, but may actually increase the milk supply.

There are two types of progesterone contraceptives besides the birth control pill that may also be used while breast feeding. The first is a progesterone injection, which is given every three months. The second involves implanting six capsules under the skin of the inner part of the upper arm. These capsules may be left in place for up to five years. Both of these methods require less effort than the pills, but are meant to be used for longer periods of time.

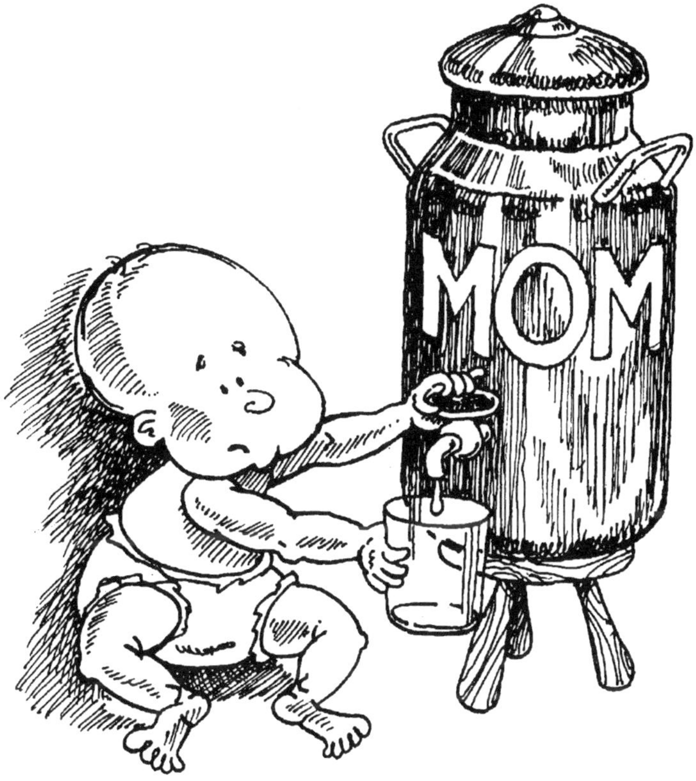

Why, you may ask, are combination birth control pills so much more popular than progesterone-only pills in non–breast feeding women? The answer is simple. The majority of non–breast feeding women on progesterone contraceptive methods have totally unpredictable bleeding, at least for the first year of use. The combination pills, on the other hand, give predictable, cyclic bleeding in most users. If there is one thing I have learned about women through the years, it's that you quickly lose their friendship if you make them bleed irregularly. When women are breast feeding, however, they rarely bleed on progesterone contraceptives.

Of course you can use the "you can't get pregnant while you're breast feeding" technique of birth control. This technique, which is addressed in the last question, is a favorite among obstetricians—or at least the ones who owe payments on their condos in Tahiti.

REFERENCES

Zacharias S, Aguilera E, Assenzo JR, Zanartu J. Effects of hormonal and non hormonal contraceptives on lactation and incidence of pregnancy. [Citation?]

Miscellaneous Myths & Facts

Finally, I leave you with Miscellaneous Myths and Facts. As the title suggests, these are all of the myths that I couldn't fit into other categories. It contains one of my all time favorite myths—the couvade. This is the concept that men actually go through some of the same symptoms as their wives during pregnancy. For those of you guys that experienced some weight gain, mood swings, and food cravings when your significant other was pregnant *(of course this never happened to me),* take special notice of this question.

QUESTION: Can men experience many of the symptoms of pregnancy their pregnant spouses are feeling?

A. Only those with a beer belly of adequate proportions.
B. No, that's absurd.
C. Yes. There is a universal condition where men actually experience nausea, weight gain, mood swings, and other symptoms right along with their partner.
D. Probably not. Some just get tired of their partners getting all of the attention.

ANSWER: C.

Many of my friends and relatives don't know this, but my undergraduate major was in anthropology. Pretty strange, huh?. Well, ever since I was a kid, I wanted to go into medicine. After graduation from high school, I entered college and like many other aspiring doctors to be I chose biology as my major. *WHAT A SNOOZER!* After a couple of quarters of learning about the wonderful world of plankton, I took a course in anthropology. For the uninitiated, this is not the study of Anthrax, but rather the study of mankind (and womankind). In particular, I was fascinated by the various cultures around the world and how incredibly different their worlds were from mine. One particular aspect of many cultures is something called the couvade. The couvade is a condition where men actually experience many of the same symptoms as their pregnant wives. These symptoms could include nausea, weight gain or loss, insomnia, emotional instability, constipation, diarrhea, headaches, toothaches, fatigue, and restlessness. In my literature search, which went back about 30 years, I found over 30 studies that addressed this issue of the couvade.

The incidence of this syndrome among men whose spouses were pregnant ranged from 11 percent to 65 percent in the various studies. Different authors offer different theories for this behavior. The most common theory involves the father-to-be's underlying anxiety about the pregnancy. He may be concerned about his ability to adapt to this impending lifestyle change, his ability to adequately support his family, or possibly failing at fatherhood. Some authors simply see the couvade as a statement of the father wanting to be recognized as an important part of the pregnancy. In any event, these men suffer physical symptoms that are derived from psychological concerns about their spouses' pregnancy and impending delivery.

The most common group of men affected by this condition are less socioeconomically advantaged working-class men who are experiencing an unwanted pregnancy. A researcher in Scandinavia named Bogren also found that men who hold their infants in their right arm are more likely to suffer from the couvade, have male infants, and identify with their mothers. *(I wonder how much he gets paid to make these earth-*

shattering revelations?) In any event, this condition seems to go beyond cultural boundaries, affecting men throughout the world. So all of you soon-to-be fathers out there, stock up on the pickles and ice cream—it could be a long nine months. For those of you who have nothing better to do but read up on weird conditions, Klein from the University of Texas at Galveston has a great review article concerning the couvade with 37 references on the subject.

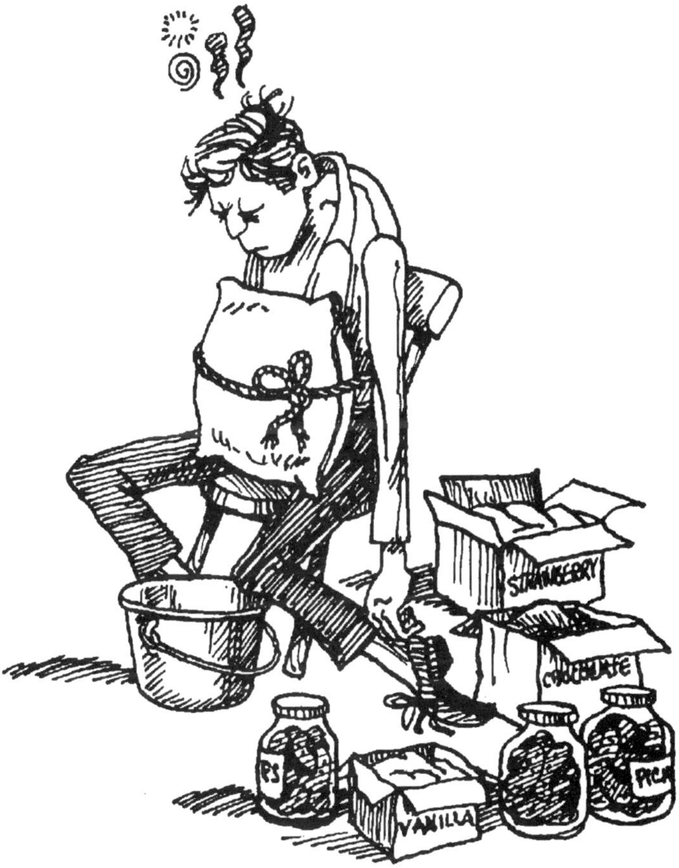

REFERENCES

Bogren LY: The couvade syndrome: background variables. *Acta Psychiatr Scand* Oct; 70(4): 316–20, 1984.

Bogren LY: The couvade syndrome and side preference in child holding. *Acta Psychiatr Scand* Mar; 7(2): 221–48, 1985.

Connor GK, Denson V: Expectant fathers' response to pregnancy: review of literature and implications for research in high-risk pregnancy. *J Perinat Neonatal Nurs* Sep; 4(2): 33–42, 1990.

Klein H: Couvade syndrome: male counterpart to pregnancy. *Int J Psychiatry* Med 21(1): 57–69, 1991.

Masoni S, Maio A, Trimarchi G, de Punzio C, Fioretti P: The couvade syndrome. *J Psychosom Obstet Gynaecol* Sep; 15(3): 125–31, 1994.

Wilson LG: The couvade syndrome. *Am Fam Physician* May; 15(5): 157–60, 1977.

QUESTION: What are stretch marks and how can they be prevented?

A. Reddish lines that develop on the abdomen of a pregnant woman as the skin is stretched during pregnancy. Prevention is possible with creams.
B. Skin markings that develop during pregnancy, but don't have anything to do with stretching. They are not preventable.
C. Skin bruises that Michael Jordan leaves on defenders as he stretches toward the basket during a basketball game. They are not preventable if you are the defender.
D. Skin marks that are a result of pregnant women bumping into things.

ANSWER: B.

It always amazes me how some women develop pink or purple bands over the abdomen, breasts, thighs, and buttocks during pregnancy, and some come through it without a mark. Equally amazing are the arrays of potions that are available to "prevent" these dreaded linear markings. What causes these to appear, and is there any evidence that they can be prevented?

Stretch marks, or striae as they are known in the medical community, are linear tears in the skin and actually have very little to do with stretching. They are probably caused by steroid hormones which are produced in great supply in pregnancy. There are actually some medical conditions where men and non-pregnant women can get these stretch marks. In these conditions steroid hormones are produced from a gland called the adrenal gland, and if the condition is not treated, stretch marks develop.

If all pregnant women have these steroid hormones, then why don't all of them develop stretch marks? It appears some women have a genetic predisposition toward developing striae and others don't. Going along with this idea, Caucasians are much more likely to develop these than are Asians and African–Americans. If there is a genetic basis for this condition, then you would think creams and oils would be useless in preventing them. This is pretty much the case. I could find two studies—one from Germany and one from Britain—that still keep all of you oil lovers' hopes alive. The study from Germany took 50 pregnant women and divided them into an oil-treated group and an untreated group. At the end of their pregnancy, one third of the oil-treated group had stretch marks, and two thirds of the untreated group had stretch marks. Moreover the group that was oiled daily was much happier. So the heck with all of the other zillion studies that poo-poo the value of skin treatments during pregnancy. All of you pregnant women who are reading this book need to stop by the local pharmacy, stock up on your favorite oils, and put your significant other to work. If those darn stretch marks start to pop up, then just get him to work harder...I won't tell.

REFERENCES

Creasy RK, Resnick, R. *Maternal-Fetal Medicine.* WB Saunders Co. Phila., Pa. p.1102, 1994.

Davey CMH: Factors associated with the occurrence of striae gravidarum. *J Obstet Gynecol Br Commonw* 70: 1113, 1972.

Poidevin LOS; Striae gravidarum: Their relationship to adrenal cortical hyperfunction. *Lancet* ii: 436, 1959.

Wierrani F, Kozak W, Schramm W, Grunberger W: [Attempt of preventive treatment of striae gravidarum using preventive massage ointment administration] *Wien Klin Wochenschr* 104(2): 42–4, 1992.

QUESTION: Are women who have small shoe sizes more likely to have a Cesarean section?

A. This is true. If more obstetricians paid attention to this fact, they could schedule Cesarean sections for these women and save them the time and trouble of a long labor.
B. It is true that smaller women have smaller feet and tend to have a higher Cesarean section rate, but clinically this information is not very useful.
C. No, this is false. In fact, women with smaller feet actually have a lower Cesarean section rate than other women.
D. You're looking at the wrong factor—it's the size of her partner that's important in determining whether junior will fit or not. Shoe size is irrelevant.

ANSWER: B.

Do any of you women out there have a pair of feet *(like mine)* that would put Godzilla to shame? You know what I mean. Some real whoppers. The kind that get you confused with pontoon boats in the summer and serve as slalom skis in the winter? Well, maybe your oversized wheels give you an unmistakable advantage in life—a reduced chance of having a Cesarean section. Actually I started thinking about this possibility roughly a year ago when the following incident occurred.

It was about 5 A.M. and I was walking from the obstetrical recovery room toward my call room. I had been up most of the night with a patient whose labor ended in a Cesarean section. The surgery was done because the baby was unable to fit through the patient's snug pelvis. As I looked up, a crowd of about a dozen family members passed me on their way to see the patient and her new arrival in recovery. A few of them expressed their appreciation to me with hand shakes and some words of thanks. As the crowd moved off toward the recovery room, an elderly woman took my arm in her hand and guided me to the side of the hallway. She looked up at me with a pleasant smile and a twinkle in her eye and said, "You know, Dr. Smith, I could have told you that Mary was going to have a Cesarean section. She only wears a size $4\frac{1}{2}$ shoe. All of the women in our family with small feet have had Cesarean sections. In fact, I have won a considerable amount of money from friends and family by predicting who would have a Cesarean section and who would not. You might pay more attention to shoes. If you did...you might be able to get more sleep." I thanked her for her information, congratulated her on her new grandson, and trudged off to my call room.

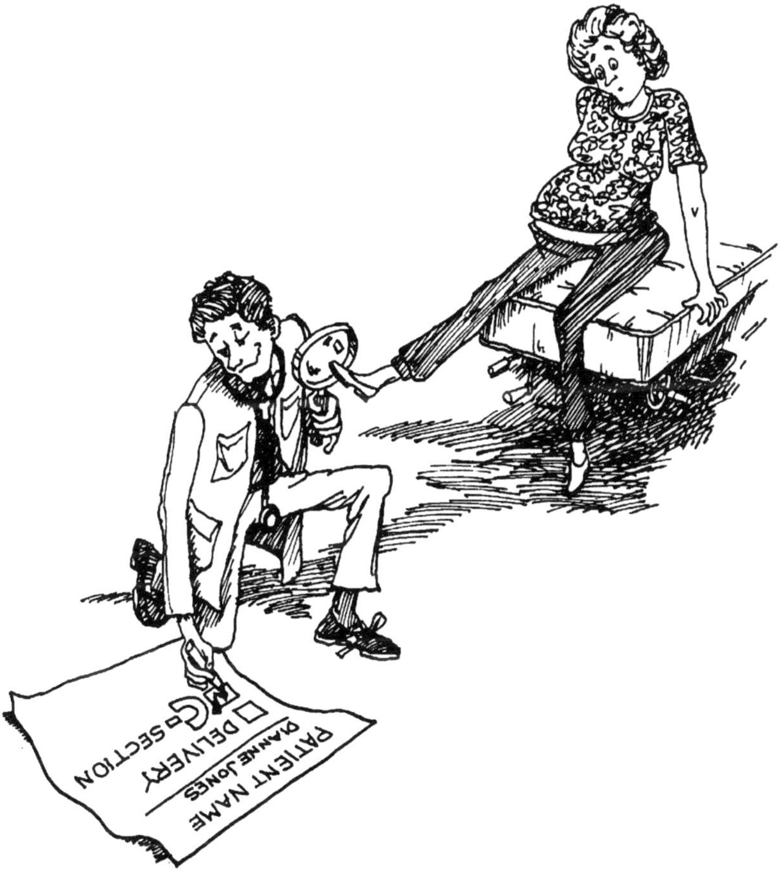

The following day, after a good night's sleep, this woman's advise kept popping into my mind. Certainly I had heard this myth before but had always blown it off as absurd. Needless to say, my curiosity got the better of me and I began researching this obscure subject. To my surprise,

I found three studies that addressed the correlation between Cesarean section rate and shoe size. In 1985, Kennedy et. al. from Hahnemann Medical College in Pennsylvania followed 76 women throughout their labor. They divided them into three groups by height and then further subdivided these groups into women with shoe sizes of greater than 5½ and those with less than 5½. Interestingly, the average birth weight of the babies born to each of these groups was the same—about seven pounds. There were five women who were less than 5 feet tall and had a shoe size of less than 5½. Three of these women (or 60 percent) ended up with a Cesarean section because the baby wouldn't fit. This was significantly higher than for any other group. The findings in this study suggested that there may be a relationship between shoe size and an increased Cesarean section rate. An obvious flaw, however, was the small sample size.

A larger British study was reported in 1985 involving 351 women. Fifty seven of these women had a shoe size of less than 4½ and an overall Cesarean section rate of 21 percent. A second group with a shoe size between 4½ and 6 had a 10 percent Cesarean section rate, and a third group with shoe sizes greater than 6 had a 1 percent rate. They concluded from this data that there was a relationship between small shoe size and an increased Cesarean section rate. Unlike the previous study, they found no correlation between height and Cesarean sections.

The latest study I found was also reported in the British literature and analyzed the height, shoe size, and Cesarean section rate of 563 women. Unlike both of the previous studies, they found no correlation between shoe size and section rate, but found a significantly higher rate in women less than 5 feet 2 inches in height. So there you have it. Out of these three studies, one found a relationship between small height, small shoe size, and an increase in Cesarean sections. One found an increased section rate in women with small shoe size but not with height, and the last found an increase with small height but not shoe size. In summary, I would have to say that women of small stature are generally at higher risk for Cesarean sections. They tend to have smaller pelvic bones and since these women don't necessarily have smaller babies than other women, their kids get stuck more often. Is this information clinically useful? Probably not. Certainly enough women have successful vaginal deliveries who are short and/or have small feet to make this information fairly useless.

REFERENCES

Frame S, Moore J, Peters A, Hall D. Maternal height and shoe size as predictors of pelvic disproportion: an assessment. *Br J Obstet Gynaecol* Dec; 92(12): 1239–45, 1985.

Kennedy JL, Greenwald E. Correlation of shoe size and obstetric outcome: an anthropometric study. *Am J Obstet Gynecol* Jun 15; 140(4): 466–7, 1981.

Mahmood TA, Campbell DM, Wilson AW. Maternal height, shoe size, and outcome of labour in white primigravidas: a prospective antropometric study. *BMJ* Aug 20–27; 297(6647): 515–7, 1988.

QUESTION: Does having heartburn during pregnancy mean your child will be born with lots of hair?

A. Sure.
B. No. That's absurd.
C. Only if he or she is a direct descendent of Romulus or Remus and is born during the full moon.
D. It depends where you're putting those antacids.

ANSWER: B.

There is a sphincter between the stomach and the esophagus (or throat) that opens and closes to let food pass from the esophagus into the stomach. This muscle opens to allow food to pass and then closes to keep the food in the stomach from going back into the esophagus. If this muscle doesn't close all of the way, acid from the stomach can escape back into the esophagus and cause a burning sensation that we call heartburn.

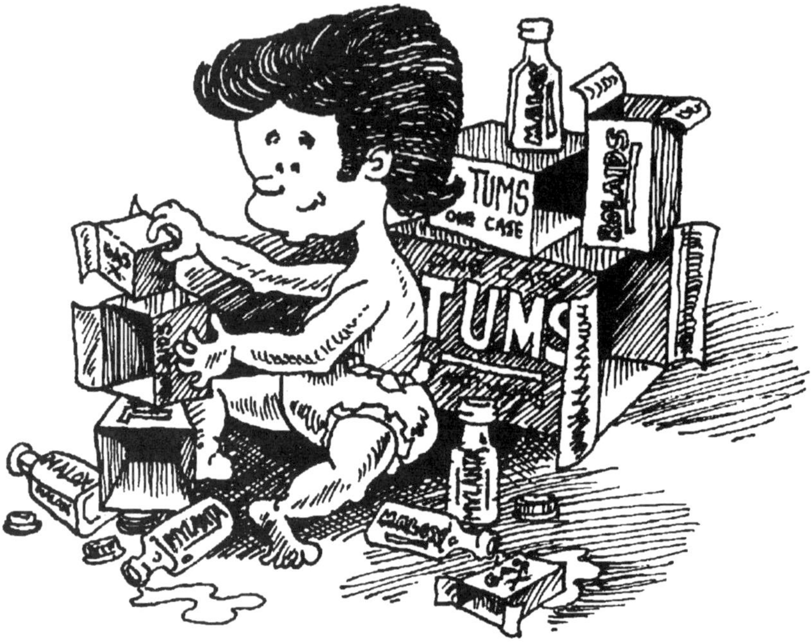

In pregnancy, a substance called progesterone is made in large quantities by the placenta. This progesterone is released into the bloodstream and relaxes all of the smooth muscle throughout the body. It so happens that the muscle between the stomach and the esophagus is made primarily of smooth muscle. This relaxing effect of progesterone on this muscle is what leads to heartburn in pregnancy.

In my experience, virtually all women experience heartburn at some time during their pregnancy. The way to improve this irritating condition is to take antacids after meals because of the large outpouring of stomach acid. At night, lying down causes the stomach acid to reflux up into the esophagus and therefore increases the heartburn, so a bedtime dose of antacids is also helpful. Another benefit of taking antacids during pregnancy is that most are a great source of calcium.

So why do some people link heartburn with having a baby with lots of hair? Beats me. Since both heartburn and having babies with a nice head of hair are common conditions, the odds of these occurring at the same time are relatively high. My guess is that some pregnant Neanderthal woman's mother-in-law made the connection way back when in a cave somewhere, and the idea stuck. Of course other theories are certainly possible.

QUESTION: How much weight should a woman gain during pregnancy?

A. As little as possible.
B. As much as she wants. This is an important issue for you guys out there. Bring up the weight thing and you're a dead man. So just leave her alone and you'll live to see another day.
C. 25 to 30 pounds, for all pregnant women regardless of their weight.
D. 15 to 40 pounds. Women who are underweight before becoming pregnant should gain more than those women who are overweight.

ANSWER: B and D. (Actually D is the right answer but you guys need to pretend that B is correct…it's for your own good).

Up until a few years ago, I would have told you 25 to 30 pounds. Why? Because I was taught in my residency that all pregnant women should gain 25 to 30 pounds during their pregnancy regardless of their pre-pregnancy weight. This was based on studies from Great Britain in the 1950s and was accepted as dogma until recently. In 1990, a committee of the National Academy of Science reviewed all of the existing data on weight gain during pregnancy and recommended a 28 to 40 pound weight gain for underweight women, 25 to 35 pounds for normal weight women, and 15 to 25 pounds for overweight women. They arrived at these figures by seeing what weight ranges yielded the best outcome in terms of having a healthy baby.

In 1992, Parker and Abrams took the recommendations by the National Academy of Science and examined 6,690 live births in the San Francisco area. They saw that the women who gained the recommended weight had normal size babies and the best outcome. Women who gained less than the recommend weight had smaller babies and, not surprisingly, women who gained more than the recommended weight had larger babies. Both the smaller and larger babies had more complications, and there was a higher Cesarean section rate for women giving birth to larger babies.

Going over recommended weight gains is all well and good, but what can the average pregnant woman do to achieve that recommended weight. Basically it is pretty simple (simple to say, that is, but not always simple to do). I tell my patients to use common sense and eat nice, well-balanced meals and avoid things like snacking on junk foods throughout the day and tossing down large desserts—two things that are extremely tempting once you get out of your first trimester. This will put you in the ball park of a normal weight gain. The last thing you want to do as a physician or a family member is to scold a woman for gaining too much weight. First of all, most pregnant women start feeling pretty depressed about their expanding body at some time in their pregnancy. Chastising women about weight gain merely has the effect of reducing them to tears and has a minimal effect on their dietary habits. Gentle reminders are much more productive in modifying overactive eating behaviors. Second of all, I despise rules that say a woman should gain a certain amount of weight per week throughout her pregnancy. It's the overall amount of weight that is important. Some women actually lose a fair amount of weight early in pregnancy do to nausea and then gain more in the last two trimesters. Other women are able to keep their weight gain more constant. When women are weighed in the office, their weight varies depending on the time of day and the clothes they are wearing. Simply put, weight gain is not important enough to ruin a woman's self-image during pregnancy (or any other time for that matter).

By the way, just how much of a woman's weight gain in pregnancy can be attributed to the baby and how much is extra weight on mom. In the average pregnancy, the baby, placenta, amniotic fluid, increased uterine weight, increased blood volume, breast enlargement, and increased "water weight" account for about 20 pounds. You guessed it. Everything else is extra. It is also true that the more children a woman has, the more weight she retains after delivery. This retained weight does not appear to be affected by the interval between deliveries or breast feeding.

In the final analysis, it is worth keeping weight gain reasonable, but let's not get too anal over this issue. This is not the time to start a restrictive diet, but a pregnant woman shouldn't feel she has free rein to eat everything in sight either. For you guys out there, cut your sweetie a little slack when she puts on a few extra pounds. She will love you for your understanding.

REFERENCES

Cunningham FG, MacDonald PC, Gant NF, Leveno KJ, Gilstrap LC. *Williams Obstetrics*. 19th edition. Appleton & Lange. Norwalk, Conn. pp. 254-55, 1993.

Parker JD, Abrams B. Prenatal weight gain advice: An examination of the recent prenatal weight gain recommendations of the Institute of Medicine. *Obstet Gynecol* 79: 664, 1992.

QUESTION: Why do twin births occur?

A. Twins are strictly genetic and always skip generations.
B. Twins arise from having intercourse twice on the same night. Identical twins come from having sex in the same position, whereas changing positions leads to nonidentical twins. (What about quads?...Could be a heck of a workout!).
C. Twins occur only when you already have more kids than you planned and you find that one in a million flawed condom right about mid-cycle.
D. Twins arise from a combination of genetic factors, as well as from man-made interventions such as fertility drugs.

ANSWER: D.

For centuries, twin births have fascinated mankind *(and womankind too—please forgive the male chauvinism).* Whether it is Romulus and Remus and the founding of Rome or Haley Mills in the *Parent Trap,* mystical twin folklore seems to pervade all cultures. Twins actually come in two varieties: 1) nonidentical or dizygotic twins and 2) identical or monozygotic twins. For simplicity, I will refer to them as nonidentical and identical twins. You may also see nonidentical twins referred to as fraternal twins.

Identical twins result when a sperm cell fertilizes an egg and as the fertilized egg grows, it splits into two identical eggs. These fertilized eggs then grow into two identical babies. Obviously then, identical twins will always be the same sex and have the same genetic make-up. The incidence of identical twins remains relatively constant in the world at a rate of about 1 in 250 births. This rate seems to be independent of age, race, geographic location, and the number of children a woman has delivered.

Nonidentical twins are another story. These twins result when two separate ovulations take place and two eggs are fertilized at the same time. These twins are no more alike than any brothers and sisters within the same family.

Nonidentical twins, unlike identical twins, show an increased incidence with age and number of deliveries. The older a woman is, and the more children she has, the more likely she is to have nonidentical twins. The father does not seem to play a big role in the inheritance of twins. There is also a large difference in nonidentical twin rates in regard to race. In the United States, white women have a rate of 1 in 100 births whereas the rate for African–American women is 1 in 79. Asian women seem to have the lowest incidence. One of the highest rates in the world is found in the Yorubas of Nigeria where 1 in 19 births result in twins! Tall women also seem to have twins more often.

Today, the single largest factor influencing the rate of nonidentical twins is the field of infertility. Drugs that aid in ovulation may increase the incidence of nonidentical twins from 5 to 40 percent depending on the drugs that are used. The newer in vitro techniques also may lead to multiple births as a number of eggs are fertilized and implanted each cycle. The majority of my patients' multiple (twins or more) pregnancies are nonidentical and result from infertility techniques.

By the way, do any of you have kids that are as infatuated with the

Parent Trap as mine are? They must have watched that movie about a thousand times. So much for twins being fascinating.

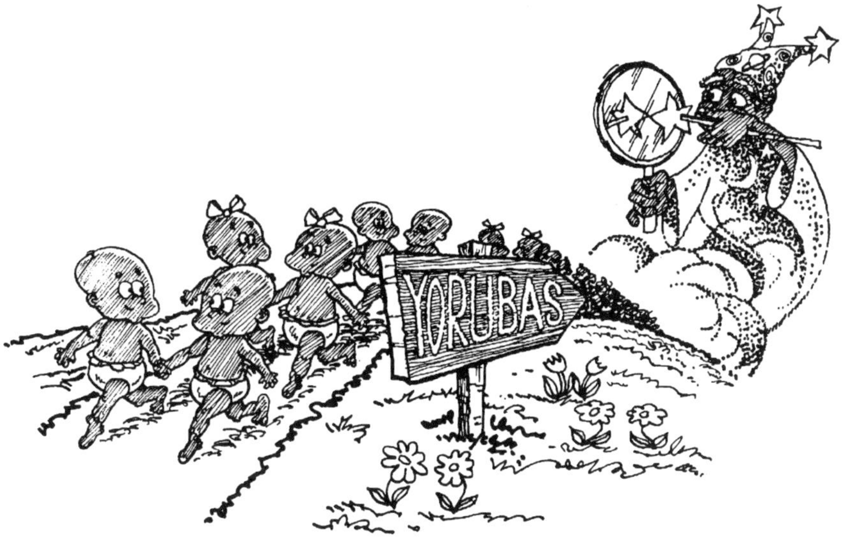

REFERENCES

Cunningham FG, MacDonald PC, Gant NF, Leveno KJ, Gilstrap LC. *Williams Obstetrics*. 19th edition. Appleton and Lange. 1993:891–894.

QUESTION: Are all babies are born with blue eyes?

A. For babies of Caucasian ancestry, this is true. Depending on genetics, the color may gradually change shortly after birth.
B. Yes. This is true for all babies.
C. No. Babies are born with the eye color that they will have for the rest of their lives.
D. This is determined predominately by your mailman's lineage.

ANSWER: A.

It was 5 A.M. and I was preparing to deliver a baby. My patient was draped and in stirrups with her husband by her side. She was pretty well exhausted from two hours of pushing, and he also looked a little rough around the edges. They seemed to have picked up their second wind, however, in anticipation of their new arrival. "Push, two, three, four, five, six, seven, eight, nine, ten," I bellowed. "Come on, you can do it! Only a few more pushes and this baby will be here!" With the next contraction, the baby's head crowned and with a mighty push, little junior was born. "Looks like a boy to me," I added and then suctioned the baby's mouth and nose after which he let out an ear piercing cry. Tears of joy rolled down the couple's faces (and even at this ungodly hour I have to admit that my eyes watered up a bit too.)

"This is what it's all about," I thought. Being able to share in these moments was what drew me into this profession. Early in my career I made a deal with myself that when my eyes stopped tearing up at deliveries and my job became routine, I would get out of OB and do something else. Here I am 17 years later doing the same thing and getting the same thrill.

My patient took the baby from my arms and laid him on her chest. Her husband put his arms around his wife and their newborn son, and they both stared lovingly into his eyes. All at once this angelic scene was interrupted by Dad's quizzical facial expression. "My son," he began, "has blue eyes." I quickly glanced at this Caucasian couple and saw that they both had dark brown eyes.

"And the mailman's eyes?" I replied. "Does anyone recall his eye color?" The couple looked at me and saw the big smile on my face. "All newborn baby's eyes are blue," I continued. Even with brown-eyed parents, they may stay blue or slowly change to a hazel or brown color later on." We all had a little chuckle and then they turned their attention back to their newborn son.

What's the deal with newborn eye color anyway? Well, the story goes like this. The part of the eye that contains the color is called the iris. The more pigment the iris contains, the darker it becomes. At birth, babies born to white couples have very little pigment, and their eyes appear bluish. Within about six months, the pigment increases in the eyes of some babies and their eyes change. If a lot of pigment is added, then their eyes become brown, and if smaller amounts are added, they may become a shade of green. If little or no pigment is added then the eyes remain blue. In babies born to couples of other racial backgrounds, this is not the case. Couples who are predominately of African–American descent, for example, usually have babies whose eyes have a large amount of pigment, giving them a rich, dark brown appearance.

What determines how much pigment will be added to the eyes of newborn babies? This is decided primarily by genetics. Let me explain this a little. You inherit one gene from your mother and one from your father, which together determine your overall eye color. As a general rule, "brown eye genes" are dominant to "blue eye genes," with green or hazel being intermediate. This means that if you inherit a brown eye gene from one parent and a blue eye gene from another, you will have brown eyes (or possibly a shade of green). Two blue-eyed parents must only have blue eye genes and will therefore only have blue-eyed kids. Looking back at the couple that I referred to at the beginning of this question, their child could end up with about anything. If each parent has a brown and a blue gene (thereby giving them brown eyes), they each could give their child their blue eye gene yielding a blue-eyed child. If both give him their brown eye gene, he will end up with brown. If he gets a brown eye gene from one parent and a blue eye gene from the other, then he will end up with brown eyes or possibly a shade of green.

In any event, eye color is determined by the amount of pigment found within the iris of the eye. The amount of pigment in the eye is determined by the parents and varies at birth, but is pretty well set by about six months of age. While the statement "all babies are born with blue eyes" may apply to one segment of the population, it varies greatly depending on ancestry. Even though I gave you some generalities in the inheritance of eye color, basing parentage on eye color is virtually impossible due to its complexity. So all of you mailmen out there can breathe a sigh of relief.

REFERENCES

Nelson WE, Behrman RE, Kliegman RM, Arvin AM. *Nelson Textbook of Pediatrics*. 15th edition. WB Saunders Co. Phila., Pa. p.1764, 1996.

O'Doherty N. *Inspecting the Newborn Baby's Eyes.* MTP Press Limited. Lancaster, England. p.12, 1986.

Tasman W, Jaeger EA. *Duane's Clinical Ophthalmology.* Lippincott-Raven Publ. Phila., Pa. (1)31 p.18, 1995.

Vaughn DG, Taylor A, Riordan-Eva P. *General Ophthalmology.* 14th edition. Appleton & Lange. Norwalk, Conn. p.28, 1995.

QUESTION: Can a newborn baby see at birth?

A. Like a hawk.
B. Like a nearsighted hawk
C. Like a bat in a blizzard
D. No, not at all.

ANSWER: C.

One of my favorite movie segments comes from the movie *Look Whose Talking* starring John Travolta, Kirstie Alley, and Bruce Willis. The birth scene where Bruce Willis gives us a blow by blow account of what it's like to be born is really a hoot. Every time I watch this birthing reenactment, I wonder to myself, "Can newborns really see that well?"

Just imagine...you have spent the only nine months of your life in total darkness inside the smallest living quarters imaginable and have been rudely expelled into the cold, bright world. You are wet and freezing your butt (and other anatomical parts) off. Mom, Dad, and Grandma are screeching annoying, cutsie noises into your ear as you attempt to open your eyes for the first time. On your first attempt to sneak a peak at the world, Aunt Susie holds something up to her face and a horrible white flash stuns you like a cattle prod. Then a big burly woman with a white outfit grabs you and starts giving you a total body massage with a towel. Just about the time you think it's okay to sneak another peak, your eyes are suddenly forced opened and some antibiotic ointment is squeezed into them. Welcome to the world!

What exactly can a newborn see in those first hours? The answer is, obviously, that nobody knows for sure. Most of the sources I found agreed that the visual acuity of a newborn is probably in the neighborhood of 20/400. This corresponds to my vision without contacts and places the infant squarely in the "can barely see your hand in front of your face" club. The infant can respond pretty well to changes in light and dark at first, but little else. One of the first objects to be recognized is mom's face during feeding. Other close up objects follow and by two weeks of age, an infant can follow a large object through an arc of 180 degrees. The child's vision steadily improves, and by 2 to 3 years his or her vision reaches the 20/30 to 20/20 range. Something else I have noticed is that although newborns tend to cry a lot, there are usually little or no tears. According to most sources, tears are not present with crying until 1 to 3 months after birth.

REFERENCES

Nelson WE, Behrman RE, Kliegman RM, Arvin AM. *Nelson Textbook of Pediatrics.* 15th edition. W B Saunder Co. Phila., Pa. p. 1764, 1996.

Postscript

Thank you for allowing me to share some of my thoughts about pregnancy with you. Hopefully, you have had a chuckle or two while gaining some insight into some of the more controversial (and not so controversial) issues in obstetrics today. As I mentioned in the Introduction, I would like to hear from those of you who have pregnancy-related questions you would like me to research and include in another edition. I am sure there are many interesting and thought-provoking topics I haven't touched.

For now, remember to keep a little humor in your life and be on the lookout for someone whose life you can brighten with some of the ideas contained in this book.

About the Author

Dr. Smith currently practices obstetrics and gynecology with two other physicians in Cincinnati, Ohio. He also is actively involved in the training of medical students and OB/GYN residents at the Good Samaritan Hospital. Dr. Smith is board-certified in obstetrics and gynecology and is a member of the Alpha Omega Alpha Honorary Medical Society, American Medical Association, Ohio State Medical Association, and the Cincinnati OB/GYN Society.

After graduating with a BA cum laude in Anthropology from the University of Cincinnati, Dr. Smith received his formal medical training at the Medical College of Ohio at Toledo. While in medical school, Dr. Smith was honored for being the top student in his class in obstetrics and gynecology as well as surgery. He completed a four-year residency in obstetrics and gynecology in Dallas, Texas before starting his clinical practice.

Dr. Smith is married and lives in Finneytown, Ohio (a small suburb of Cincinnati) with his wife Janet, three children (Ryan, Eric, and Lindsay), two dogs (Dolby and CD), a rabbit (BB), and a cockatiel named Millet.

Glossary

amenorrhea: the lack of menstrual periods.

amniocentesis: placing a needle into the uterus of a pregnant woman and drawing off amniotic fluid to obtain cells that reveal the genetic make-up of the fetus.

amniotic fluid: fluid which surrounds the baby during pregnancy. It contains liquid produced by the fetal membranes and fetal urine.

anorexia nervosa: a physical and psychological condition where individuals deprive themselves of calories in the belief that they are overweight, even in the face of extreme weight loss. Untreated, it may lead to death.

anteverted uterus: about 80 percent of all women have a uterus of this type which curves forward toward the abdomen.

artificial insemination: placing a semen sample either in the vagina or uterus for the purpose of conceiving.

aspartame: the generic name for the sweetener whose brand name is Nutrasweet.

Aunt Susie: a mythical character representing all of the women in your life who ever gave you advice you didn't really need.

birth control pills: pills which women may take to fool their body into thinking they are pregnant. This suppresses ovulation and greatly decreases the chances of becoming pregnant with intercourse.

bladder: hollow muscular organ which stores the urine produced by the kidneys. During urination, it contracts, forcing the urine through the urethra and out of the body.

breast binders: cloth wraps which apply pressure to the breasts to decrease engorgement.

breech: when the fetus has its buttocks or legs down against the cervix instead of the head.

bromocriptine: a medication previously used to decrease breast milk production and breast engorgement in women who did not wish to breast feed after delivery. It is no longer used for this purpose.

castor oil: oil derived from an African plant, which is usually used as a laxative.

cervix: the bottom part of the uterus through which the baby passes during delivery. It is also a potential area for cancer to develop. Pap smears sample the cells from the cervix to detect early precancerous changes.

Cesarean section: delivering a baby through an abdominal incision when a vaginal delivery is not possible or not desired.

chromosomes: the structures that house our genes. We normally have 46—half from our mother and half from our father. Certain medical conditions may result in a person having either extra chromosomes or not enough, leading to physical and/or mental abnormalities.

conception: the point in time when the egg and sperm meet and fertilization takes place.

congenital: present at birth. For instance, congenital birth defects are physical abnormalities that are present at birth.

couvade: the development of pregnancy-related symptoms in a male when his partner is pregnant.

diabetes mellitus: high blood sugar that develops due to a relative lack of a hormone called insulin.

dilatation and curettage: a surgical procedure that involves dilating the cervix with a series of progressively larger probes, followed by the scraping of the internal surface of the uterus to remove tissue.

Down's syndrome: a genetic condition in which the affected individual has three 21st chromosomes. Physical characteristics include a relatively small head, flat nasal bridge, eyes which appear widely spaced, and a tongue which appears large for the mouth. Heart, gastrointestinal, and other abnormalities may be present. Mental impairment ranges from minimal to severe. The occurrence of this increases with increasing age of the mother.

eclampsia: a hypertensive condition of pregnancy leading to seizures of the mother.

ectopic pregnancy: a pregnancy which develops outside the uterus. The most common type is a tubal pregnancy where the embryo implants and begins growing in the uterine tube. Removal of the embryo or tube is usually necessary to prevent tubal rupture and internal bleeding.

effacement: thinning out of the cervix.

egg: a microscopic cell that is released from a woman's ovary. This cell contains half the genetic material needed to create an embryo. The sperm cell, which contains the other half, joins with the egg in a process called fertilization.

ejaculate: the expulsion of semen from the penis during orgasm.

embryo: the name given to a developing baby from the time of conception until about eight weeks of pregnancy.

endometriosis: a condition where cells that normally line the uterus are found outside the uterus (i.e. the ovary, bowel, etc.) and continue to bleed on a monthly basis. This may lead to pelvic pain and infertility in some women.

epidural anesthesia: a type of anesthesia commonly used to provide pain relief during labor and delivery. It involves placing anesthetic medication into the space around the spinal canal through a catheter placed into the lower back. Vaginal deliveries and Cesarean sections may be performed under this type of anesthesia.

estimated date of confinement: another way of saying "due date." This is approximately 40 weeks from a woman's last menstrual period.

estrogen: a hormone produced by a woman's ovary. It is needed for ovulation.

external version: pushing on a woman's abdomen in a circular motion to change the position of a fetus into the head down position. This is usually done under ultrasound guidance.

fertilization: the process of an egg and sperm cell joining together (physically and genetically) to become an embryo.

fetal membranes: the thin layer that lines the uterine cavity and contains the fetus and amniotic fluid.

fetal monitor: a device which records the fetal heart rate and uterine contractions while a woman is in labor. It may also be used prenatally to detect fetal distress or to aid in the diagnosis of labor.

fetus: the name given to a developing baby from eight weeks after conception until delivery.

fibroids: benign muscular tumors of the uterus.

folic acid: a vitamin that when taken prenatally has been linked with a decrease in neural tube defects of the fetus.

fundal height: the distance between a pregnant woman's pubic bone and the top of her uterus. This distance in centimeters matches the number of weeks that she has completed in her pregnancy. So a woman at 28 weeks of pregnancy should have a fundal height of 28 centimeters.

genes: structures found in all of our cells that act as the blueprint for our body. They contain the information that determines what every cell in our body does.

general anesthesia: inducing a sleep-like state in a patient by placing medication through an intravenous line, followed by having the patient breathe an anesthetic gas. This state is achieved just prior to and during surgical procedures to keep the patient free of pain. The anesthetic agents are withdrawn upon completion of the procedure.

gestational diabetes mellitus: high blood sugar that some women develop during pregnancy.

gynecology: the branch of medicine that deals with caring for women and their medical needs exclusive of pregnancy.

heartburn: an uncomfortable sensation in the middle of the chest due to the reflux of stomach acid into the lower esophagus.

hemorrhoids: dilated rectal veins, which may become more dilated during pregnancy and delivery, causing discomfort and bleeding.

hormone: a substance produced by a gland (such as the ovary or testicle) and released into the bloodstream to cause an effect somewhere else in the body.

human chorionic gonadotropin: a hormone put out by the placenta during pregnancy. This hormone is detected in pregnancy tests and is responsible for many symptoms of early pregnancy including nausea and breast tenderness.

hypertension: high blood pressure.

hysterectomy: a surgical procedure to remove the uterus.

infertility: a condition which exists when a couple has unprotected intercourse for one year without achieving a pregnancy.

insulin: a hormone which is responsible for getting sugar from the bloodstream into the cells of the body.

intercourse: the penetration of the vagina by the erect penis, which may lead to the release of semen containing sperm cells into the vagina.

in vitro fertilization: removing an egg from the ovary, fertilizing it with a sperm cell, and then placing the resulting embryo into the uterus to grow. Usually more than one embryo is used to increase the chances of fertilization.

iris: the part of the eye which contains pigment and gives the eye its color.

labor: contractions of the uterus that force the fetus downward and lead to the birth of a baby

letdown reflex: ejection of milk from the breast caused by oxytocin, which is released from an area in the brain called the pituitary gland. This accounts for the leakage a woman may get when she hears her hungry baby cry.

lightening: a downward movement of the baby into the pelvis that may occur long before labor starts, just prior to labor, or not at all.

meconium: greenish-colored amniotic fluid which results when a fetus has a bowel movement before birth.

menses: the vaginal bleeding that occurs when a pregnancy is not achieved and the lining of the uterus is sloughed off.

menstrual cycle: the continuous building up of the lining of the uterus followed by sloughing when a pregnancy is not achieved. This cyclic building and sloughing is referred to as the menstrual cycle.

mini-pill: a type of birth control pill that contains only progesterone and is commonly used while breast feeding.

miscarriage: lay term for the loss of a pregnancy before 20 weeks of gestation.

mucous plug: sticky material found within the cervical canal. It may become dislodged and exit from the vagina prior to labor or remain until labor starts.

multipara: a woman who has given birth to more than one child.

neural tube defect: an abnormality of the fetus involving the brain or spinal cord. Spina bifida is an example where a portion of the spinal cord is left uncovered and exposed.

nipple stimulation test: stimulating the nipples during pregnancy to produce uterine contractions. The fetal heart rate pattern is monitored during these contractions to see if the fetus is in distress.

obstetrics: the branch of medicine that deals with pregnancy and the birth of a baby.

oral contraceptives: see birth control pills.

orgasm: involuntary muscular contractions that occur in the male around the time of ejaculation, and in the female after sexual stimulation.

osteoporosis: the loss of calcium from bone tissue leading to brittle bones that fracture easily.

ovulation: the time during a woman's cycle when an egg is released from the ovary.

oxytocin: a hormone produced in the pituitary gland in the brain. It is responsible for ejecting milk from the nipple during breast feeding and for maintaining uterine contractions during labor. See Pitocin.

pap smear: sampling the cells of the cervix during a pelvic exam to detect precancerous or cancerous cells.

pelvic exam: exam which evaluates the female reproductive tract (the vulva, vagina, cervix, uterus, uterine tubes and ovaries).

pelvis: a bony structure that houses the uterus, tubes, ovaries, and bladder. The baby is forced by the uterus through the pelvic canal during delivery.

Pitocin: the brand name of synthetically manufactured oxytocin. This hormone may be used intravenously to initiate labor or to strengthen inadequate contractions during labor.

placebo: a medication that is devoid of any action. For example, placebo birth control pills allow a woman to continue taking pills during her week of bleeding when no oral hormone is needed. This keeps her in the habit of taking a pill every day.

placenta: a disc-like organ about the size of a Frisbee. One side is attached to the uterine wall and the other to the baby by an umbilical cord. It provides the baby with nutrients from the mother and removes fetal waste products by a unique filtering process.

placental abruption: a pulling away of the placenta from the uterine wall that can interrupt the oxygen and food supply to the fetus.

postpartum: after delivery. For example, the office visit which occurs six weeks after delivery is called the six-week postpartum visit.

preeclampsia: a condition which develops during pregnancy where a woman's blood pressure becomes elevated. It is usually associated with a release of protein in the urine and symptoms such as headache and blurred vision.

pregnancy-induced hypertension: high blood pressure that develops as a consequence of pregnancy.

premature delivery: delivery of an infant before he or she has reached full maturity. (Note that this is based on the maturity of the baby and not on the weeks of gestation).

premature labor: uterine contractions leading to the delivery of an infant before he or she has reached full maturity. (Note that this is based on the maturity of the baby and not on the weeks of gestation).

premature rupture of membranes: rupture of the fetal membranes before the onset of contractions regardless of the age of the infant.

prenatal: before birth, as in prenatal exam or prenatal visit.

preterm delivery: delivery of an infant prior to 38 weeks. (Note that this is based on the weeks of gestation and not on the maturity of the baby).

preterm labor: uterine contractions leading to a downward movement of the baby thereby changing the cervix prior to 38 weeks. (Note that this based on the weeks of gestation and not on the maturity of the baby).

preterm premature rupture of membranes: rupturing of the fetal membranes before 38 weeks gestation.

primipara: a woman who has given birth to one child.

progesterone: a hormone produced by a woman's ovary and also by the placenta during pregnancy. It is needed to maintain a normal pregnancy.

promethazine: an anti-nausea medication that is commonly used in pregnancy. It comes in tablet, injectable, and suppository forms and goes by the brand name Phenergan.

prostaglandins: hormones found in many tissues including the uterus and fetal membranes. They are probably responsible for initiating labor and causing cramps during periods.

quickening: the time during a pregnancy when a woman first feels the baby move.

rad: a unit of measure of radiation exposure (x-rays).

retroverted uterus: a normal uterine position where the uterus is tilted backward. About 20 percent of all women have a uterus oriented in this position.

sac: the membranes around the baby and amniotic fluid. This can be visualized on ultrasound early in pregnancy.

sacrum: the lower part of the spinal column from which the coccyx or "tailbone" hangs. This forms the back wall of the pelvis.

semen: a mixture of sperm cells and fluid from the prostate gland. This is the proper name for the fluid that is expelled from the penis during intercourse.

sex: refers to the male or female gender or to the act of intercourse.

siblings: children born to the same parents.

sperm: microscopic cells similar in appearance to tadpoles. They are made in the testicles of the male and released during ejaculation. One of these cells may combine with an egg resulting in fertilization. Sperm cells contain half the genetic material needed to create an embryo. The egg contains the other half.

sperm antibodies: substances produced by a woman that can attack sperm cells in the vagina and immobilize them, leading to infertility.

steroids: hormones (either synthetic or natural) derived from cholesterol that have many functions throughout the body. The sex steroids estrogen, progesterone, and testosterone are examples.

stretch marks: reddish lines that can develop on the abdomen (and sometimes the hips, thighs, and breasts) of pregnant women.

term pregnancy: when a pregnancy progresses to 38 to 42 weeks.

toxemia: an older term for preeclampsia used when it was thought this hypertensive condition of pregnancy was caused by a toxic substance within the body. The true cause is unknown today.

transverse lie: when the fetus is lying sideways in the uterus instead of head down.

trimester: one third of a pregnancy. Each trimester is described by the terms first, second, or third trimester and lasts a little over 13 weeks.

tubal pregnancy: the most common type of ectopic pregnancy. See ectopic pregnancy.

twins: two children born to the same parents during the same pregnancy. They may be identical (derived from the same embryo) or nonidentical (from different embryos).

ultrasound: using sound waves to produce an image of a fetus on a small TV-like screen. These images are used to date a pregnancy and study the anatomy of the fetus and placenta. Ultrasounds are also used to study other organs such as the gallbladder, heart, and breasts.

umbilical cord: long blood vessels that run from the fetal abdomen to the placenta. These vessels transfer oxygen and nutrients from the mother (via the placenta) to the developing fetus. Fetal waste products are transferred back to the mother so that her body can dispose of them.

uterus: the muscular organ that serves as a temporary dormitory for a fetus. During labor it contracts to expel the newborn infant.

vagina: smooth, pliable tube-like structure between the cervix and vulva which accommodates the penis during intercourse and dilates to allow passage of the fetus during delivery.

vena cava: the large vein that brings blood low in oxygen from the lower part of the body back to the heart.

visual acuity: how well someone can see.

vulva: the outer, visible genitalia of a woman including the labia majora, labia minora, and the clitoris.

wean: to discontinue breast feeding.

Index

A

B

C

D

E

F